Insight **Yoga**

INSIGHT YOGA

Sarah Powers

Foreword by Paul Grilley

Photography by Matthew Carden

 SHAMBHALA · BOSTON & LONDON · 2008

Shambhala Publications, Inc.
Horticultural Hall
300 Massachusetts Avenue
Boston, Massachusetts 02115
www.shambhala.com

9 8 7 6 5 4 3
Printed in the United States of America

⊗ This edition is printed on acid-free paper that meets the American
National Standards Institute z39.48 Standard.

♻ This book was printed on 30% postconsumer recycled paper. For
more information please visit www.shambhala.com.

Distributed in the United States by Random House, Inc.,
and in Canada by Random House of Canada Ltd

Library of Congress Cataloging-in-Publication Data
Powers, Sarah.
Insight yoga / Sarah Powers; foreword by Paul Grilley;
photography by Matthew Carden.—1st ed.
p.   cm.
Includes bibliographical references and index.
ISBN 978-1-59030-598-0 (pbk.: alk. paper)
1. Yoga. I. Title.
RA781.7.P69 2008
613.7'046—dc22
2008017296

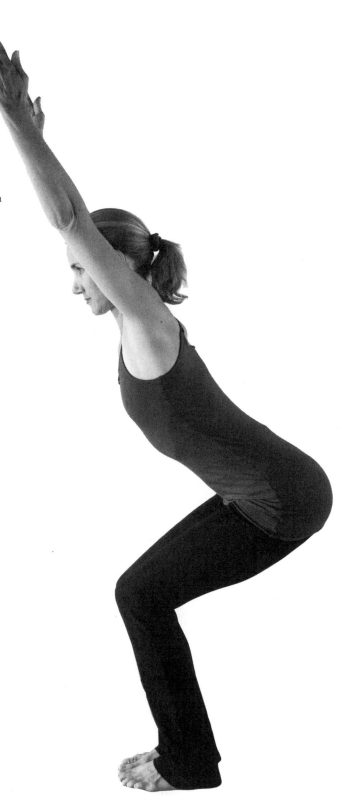

For my mother, whose creative and impassioned writing style
taught me about the beauty of words.
And to my eldest brother Conrad, who introduced me to yoga.

Contents

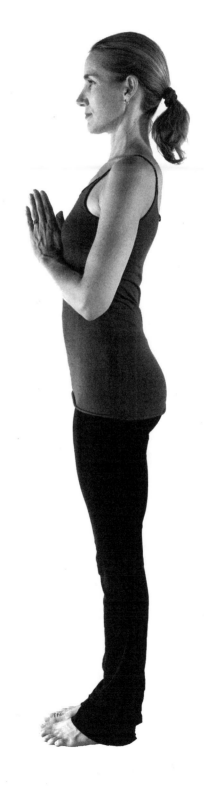

Foreword

To borrow a phrase from George Martin, Sarah Powers is like the Beatles: she has been talented from the beginning, but we had no idea how good she would get. Sarah has been blessed with beautiful features and a skeleton suited for elegant postures. It is only natural that her image has graced the covers of yoga magazines and conference posters. It seems almost unfair that she is also scholarly by nature, a constant reader, a diligent practitioner, and a humble student of any teaching she encounters. And now we, her readers, discover that she is a lucid writer as well.

Modern people want to know why—"Why should kings rule?" "Why should I do as the Church commands?" "Why does the apple fall?" To be sure, all peoples have asked questions of their existence, but most were satisfied with answers given in their holy texts or traditions. Modern people question all traditions; in fact, they mistrust them. It is the modern dharma to build up new traditions of science, medicine, and religion based on explicable, reproducible, testable principles.

Yoga has historically been called the "science of sciences." If it is to remain true to its calling, it must rebuild itself along modern scientific lines. Until recently this would have been very hard to do, because its ancient theories were based on descriptions of energy centers and channels in the body that science had not recognized. But thanks to the work of people like Dr. Hiroshi Motoyama, Dr. Yoshio Manaka, Dr. James Oschman, and many others, we are rediscovering the truth behind these ancient theories. And now Sarah Powers has created a practical manual of yoga based on these new/old yogic principles.

What are chakras? How do they affect us? What is chi? Prana? How do yoga postures affect our health? Our emotions? Our thoughts? What are meridians? Are acupuncture and yoga related? How do asanas affect meditation? How does meditation affect asanas? Sarah's book is a personal, concise, and clear response to all of these questions.

A yoga book should be personal. A medical book doesn't have to be personal, and a mathematics book isn't personal. This is because the outcomes of these sciences are external and measurable by impersonal scales. But the fruits of spiritual practice are subjective; indeed, the spiritual path is *the* subjective experience. Science can measure brain waves and heart rates, but a yogi's truest test is inward calm and deeper spiritual understanding. The Sanskrit word for the testimony of a spiritual practitioner is *agama* (direct perception or report). Unlike in the case of a math book, if a book on yoga did not possess a personal element, I would view it with suspicion.

Sarah's book is a yoga book. It is not merely Taoist or Buddhist or Sanskrit. It embodies what the term *yoga* has historically stood for: a system of practices that cultivates all levels of a human being. Sarah employs Taoist terms, Buddhist terms, and Sanskrit terms, depending on which most clearly and succinctly describe the underlying ideas. It is a historical accident that Chinese Taoists elaborated certain energetic ideas better than others, that the Tibetan Buddhists elaborated subtler mental processes, and that the Sanskrit peoples elaborated deeper inner and outer cosmologies. All these systems describe aspects of reality that were most pertinent to them at the time of their creation. This is much like a medical doctor using Latin words to describe anatomy, chemical terms to describe physiology, and German words to describe psychology.

Sarah has written a yoga book that is true to her experience while avoiding sectarian claims of privilege for any tradition. It is her readers who benefit from this honest effort. I sincerely hope that by reading Sarah's text all yoga students will find clarification of their practice, no matter what their professed style.

Paul Grilley

Insight **Yoga**

I

What Is Yoga?

Yoga can be understood as a set of behaviors that develops a holistic experience of the body, heart, and mind. It is a process of fully inhabiting ourselves and our life in a radically engaging and inquisitive way. Through this training we develop a healthy capacity to literally take up residence in our bodies and minds, which can then lead us into simple presence. Presence is a quality of being that is open and aware. This body-mind presence serves as the ground for compassion and wisdom to emerge within us.

Although there are many branches of yoga, the philosophy can be defined as a joining or yoking (the translation of *yoga*) of the many seemingly opposing layers of our being—mind and body, inner with outer, activity with receptivity, subject with object—the result of which is a nondual or inclusive state of mind in which we are able to experience the challenging dualities of life without falling into dualism. Dualism is a state of mind in which we sever a piece of experience from the integral whole and subsequently see it as independent and separate.

The fruition of a committed yoga practice is the capacity to deeply relax the inner struggle with life's paradoxes. Someone who is steeped in yoga is better able to tolerate the extremes of heat or cold, agility or immobility, sadness or joy, free from psychological confusion, resistance, or struggle. A yoga practitioner learns to question the assumption that we are separate from what we experience and must therefore strive to accumulate and hold on to that which is pleasant and comforting, while seeking to avoid and rid ourselves of that which is unpleasant, difficult, or threatening.

The path of yoga, although diverse, is a set of practices that moves us out of comfort zones in our bodies and minds, engendering the possibility of broadening our capacity for connection and inclusion. This process becomes possible by learning to dwell inside our bodies and minds with kind yet keen observance coupled with intimate participation. We learn to be fully engaged in feeling our bodies and mental states in various poses and contemplations, as well as to observe how we are responding to our moment-to-moment experience as it unfolds. A yoga practice is therefore an in-depth training in participatory observation and enhancement of the body, heart, and mind.

In body-centered yoga practices, we move our body into poses (asanas) that shape our bones and tissues into certain patterns. This helps properly move the inner animating force or energy body, aiding our natural vitality. The idea in yoga is that there is a whole universe of experience occurring in the unseen realm of existence, which is constantly influencing us. Because we cannot reach out and literally touch this aspect of life, we are often unaware of its existence, or our saturation in it. This energetic dimension, often called prana by the Indians or chi by the Chinese, animates all life.

The reason it is essential to learn about and direct this vital energy within us is because its quality and mobility through our bodies immediately impacts how we feel physically, emotionally, and mentally. Therefore, strengthening the energy body and enhancing its mobility enhances not only our health, but also our potential for deeper states of mind. For this to occur, we need to carve out regular times to practice yoga and meditation. In addition to going to classes, developing a home practice teaches us how to maintain our own interest in self-discovery. This private time spent going inward begins to ignite an attitude of inner investigation throughout our day. We start to see that yoga can be an inward journey of body-mind sensitivity during both our so-called practice time and our time spent everywhere else. It is at this point that yoga is no longer relegated to an activity we do while wearing certain clothes at the yoga center or gym, but instead becomes a living vehicle for embodied wholeness, a potent path of transformation.

Yoga as a Path of Self-Transformation

The classical term for "path" is *marga* in Sanskrit. In Buddhist texts it refers to the way or path pointed out by the Buddha that leads to a life of awareness and an escape from the misery of a deluded existence. If we think of "home" as a state of mind free from a life wrought with despair and disconnection, then a "path" leads us home.

A path can be thought of in many ways. Buddhist scholar Stephen Batchelor often points out that it is both a noun and a verb, simultaneously meaning a clearing that allows free movement

and that movement itself (as in to "path" along the clearing). As Tenzin Palmo relates in her teachings about Tibetan Buddhism, a path can also be thought of as the winding ascension up a steep mountain. As we first ascend, the climb feels steep and unforgiving; our naive enthusiasm easily wears thin and we often look for a reason to abandon our commitment altogether. We may feel unsure if we are even on the right road, wondering if we have what it takes to make the journey. And then, suddenly, we round a corner and get an unexpected glimpse of the summit. The goal is still far away, but we now know this road will lead us there.

As we "path" on our journey in search of true liberation, the clouds of forgetfulness may shroud our motivation. Still, we continue to persevere, moving along on the wings of faith that our brief glimpses of insight have given us. It is at this point that we move from an ordinary life with some yoga thrown in for health benefits to a sincere commitment to live an authentic life devoted to remaining inside awareness, whatever obstacles we may encounter. This can be thought of as a commitment to living our lives in a nonresistant flow with ourselves and the world around us. It is at this point that our "pathing" becomes yoga.

But we don't always know where to start on the path. How do we move from taking a few yoga classes once in a while to living lives dedicated to awareness? In both Tibetan and Indian yoga we must engage in three levels of development in order to inhabit a true spiritual path. The first step engages the intellect. We must educate ourselves about self-exploration through the teachings of others, whether we hear these teachings directly (which is preferable), read about them, or both. The second step engages the mind and heart. We contemplate what we have learned, wrestling with the material by ruminating over it, continually reflecting on what makes sense to us and what provokes questions. We need to at least understand the basic tenets of a path and be intrigued by the questions it raises before we can go to the next phase. The third and final step requires a commitment of our whole being. We must sincerely take up the practices themselves, with clear understanding of their purpose, methods, and potential short- and long-term effects. An ancient yogic adage from the Upanishads sheds some light on this process: "Understanding without practice is better than practice without understanding. Understanding with practice is better than understanding without practice. Resting in our authentic nature is better than any understanding or practice."

For all three levels to be navigated skillfully, we need to spend time with teachers. Books, while not substitutes for face-to-face experience, can be used as complementary reinforcement to help us stay on track. Finding an appropriate teacher whose language and methods are in sync with our constitution and level of development is a crucial initial stage on our path. Whether we find teachers through reading their books, hearing about them from friends, or shopping around at the local yoga and/or Buddhist center, we must eventually commit ourselves to thoroughly investigating what a particular teacher has to offer and be willing to apply his or her teachings in our own practice.

Teachers can act as invaluable guides to our own path by teaching us new ways of thinking, behaving, and being. They encourage honesty, integrity, and inquiry, while helping us deal skillfully with the obstacles we encounter, such as our inevitable physical limitations, negative emotional afflictions, and mental distortions. Teachers help us navigate stormy seas when we might easily drown on our own, and they encourage us to stay with our practice when we might otherwise give up or become distracted by and attached to accomplishments along the way. The teachers with whom we choose to spend time do not need to be fully enlightened; they just need to be a few steps ahead of us regarding the aspects of the path we are learning from them. Although we may need to abandon certain teachers and adopt others along our journey, our teachers will continue to act as our spiritual friends and mentors, helping us to deepen our capacity to listen to our own essential nature.

Yogic Cosmology

Both Indian and Chinese yogis suggest that all manifest reality stems from an unseen universal force of infinite expansiveness that is without beginning or end, a singular pulsation or unmoving center from which all action springs. It is thought of as the sum total of the universe and beyond, and it literally refers to the power behind all form. This primordial principle is referred to as Brahman by Hindus, the Tao by Taoists, and Sunyata by Buddhists. Each tradition describes this ineffable concept in unique ways, but all three agree (more or less) that the dimension of infinite energy is the genesis of creation itself and is often expressed as being seated in the human heart.

Yogic cosmology describes existence as a display of three "worlds" emanating out from the infinite expanse, or universal force. The coarsest and most obvious is the physical reality of form. It consists of everything we can know through our sense organs, including the earth and all its formations, as well as our body with its fluids and bones, tissues, organs, muscles, and skin. This manifold dimension's underlying characteristic is change, as all things that come into being continually go through multiple metamorphoses and then ultimately dissolve. It is called the *annamaya kosha* (*kosha* means "sheath" or "layer") and refers to our form body.

The second level of existence is our personal intermediary between the universal formless reality and our intimate experience on the physical level. This is the pranic body, which exists in a subtle, formless dimension but has a direct impact on form. It is experienced through subtle feeling (best described as an energetic, felt sense), intuition, imagination, and visualization. It is the realm of energy and cannot be understood through concrete methods of reasoning; it can only be known through direct experience. It is a kind of mental double of the physical world explored for thousands of years by inner seekers from all the wisdom traditions. This is the domain of the subtle body, sometimes called the psyche or soul, which is dependent on the physical system for the input of experience. It acts as a mediator between the physical world and the more formless abstract levels of our being. All manifest existence has this subtle double, but it is humans with our more advanced brains who can be aware of while simultaneously dwelling within this subtle body.

Developing an understanding of this energetic dimension frees us from being solely identified with the mercurial physical dimension. As we develop an awareness of the subtle body, we may start to loosen our fear-based attachment to our physical experience and begin to recognize our true estate, our essential, unbound nature. This subtle body sheath is described as having three refined layers called the *pranamaya kosha* (energy body), *manomaya kosha* (mind sheath) and *vijnanamaya kosha* (consciousness).

The third dimension is even more elusive than the subtle body. It is free of form, color, and gender, and it is called the *anandamaya kosha,* or causal body; it is a dimension of pure potential energy, the innermost source of our existence, often called the spirit. It is not quantifiable in any meaningful way but acts as a precursor to all subtle and physical form. It is a functional blueprint of all possibility. The healing modalities of Indian Ayurveda, Tibetan medicine, and Taoist Chinese medicine all stem from an understanding that our human existence unfolds within these three dimensions.

Typically we are unaware when we begin a yoga practice that we have vast reservoirs of energy and aliveness lying dormant within us. We often assume our bodies should function well without much caring attention or proper fuel. Through a skillful yoga practice coupled with a healthy diet, we can become much healthier. Initially we will notice positive changes just by moving our body in ways we never used to, and eventually change occurs because we become more attuned to our breathing, energy rhythms, mind states, and innermost potential.

As we develop a yoga practice involving postures, breath work, and meditation, understanding some principles of Taoism and Chinese medicine can help deepen our relationship with ourselves in our daily practice. My personal experience on the yogic path became much more meaningful as I began to understand the intersection between yoga, Chinese medicine, and Buddhism.

2

My Personal Journey

I HAVE PRACTICED YOGA now for more than twenty years, and my love for the practice has only grown stronger with each footprint I've made on the path. My interest began as a young adult, when I would ruminate over what constituted a meaningful life. I began feeding my hunger for meaning intellectually, reading everything from William Butler Yeats to Carl Jung, Carlos Casteneda to Ken Wilber, and Suzuki Roshi to Dilgo Khyentse Rinpoche.

Even though I was unclear about what I wanted to be when I grew up, I decided I would get a graduate degree in transpersonal psychology in order to unite my interest in Western-based psychotherapeutic understanding with the Eastern meditative traditions I was reading about. A year into the program, I concluded it was time to actually do something with my body, heart, and mind. I could no longer simply read and write papers about it. I was ready to begin a regular spiritual practice and knew I wanted one that both delved into the body and trained the mind.

It was the mideighties, and I was living in Los Angeles, where yoga popularity was just beginning to blossom. On my first day at the yoga center, I was delighted that the class was small; there were only two other people, one of whom was my husband, Ty. We had already been living together for several years and loved reading aloud from many esoteric books on the nature of reality, but we had not met any teachers or been to classes yet. Since we had both been pretty athletic all of our lives, we naively assumed this new commitment to body-mind training would come naturally and be easy for us.

I had no idea how basic and unsophisticated my awareness was until I was given gentle but precise hands-on adjustments and cues for every pose I attempted. I was astonished to find it was overwhelmingly rigorous work for my body, while my mental attention strained to keep up. Even though I felt stimulated by the challenge, I remember vowing never to return. I impatiently assumed that the only recourse was to find another system to study. Thankfully I stayed until the end, when we were given a just reward: nap time.

With an angelic voice, the teacher guided us into a state of deep relaxation in which my humiliation, sweat, and tears were soothingly melted into an unfamiliar shift in consciousness. It was while lying in the restful pose called Corpse Pose (Savasana), that I had a short but life-changing glimpse of what being vibrantly alive really meant. I recognized it as a deeply quiet absence of longing. The usual self-centered needs and wants that chronically motivated my inner world were temporarily in abeyance. I felt deeply at ease and yet fully awake for the first time.

Of course, this was merely a temporary release of me-ness. Soon after class, my familiar inner chatter reinstated its dominance over the innocence of inner quietude, but that was okay. I didn't expect it to be otherwise and was simply thankful for the gift. This brief plunge into tranquillity had drenched me to the core. I now knew it was possible to feel fully content and undivided within myself. I sensed that a regular yoga practice could be an invaluable tool for radically opening my body and mind, for helping me see my habits of conditioning, and for preparing the ground for true understanding and insight.

Becoming a Yoga Student

Over the next few years, my devotion to yoga as a transformative vehicle caused me to seek out dedicated teachers from a number of backgrounds. I was interested in finding various tools to assist me on my journey. I soon discovered that I needed to dedicate myself to a certain teaching style in order to fully integrate these new principles and practices into my life. I also recognized that there were many disciplines to choose from, and if I was going to devote myself to a sincere practice, I would have to find the teachings that were appropriate for my constitution and disposition. This was initially a daunting task.

I discovered that no one path fully addressed my many interests. Some were intensely focused on body attunement, which I now loved, but did not seem to address the heart and mental attitude. Others were directed toward training and taming the mind, but seemed to ignore harmonizing and inhabiting the body. I began to recognize that I might need to draw from a number of styles and lineages to feel nourished on many levels.

When I began practicing yoga postures regularly, I gravitated toward the physical practices

of Ashtanga and Iyengar yoga, but I occasionally enjoyed a Yin practice as well. Having begun these disciplines while still quite young, I came to them with the lethal combination of a bendy back mixed with unbridled enthusiasm to try new things. One morning, a senior yoga teacher instructed us to come into Headstand (Sirsasana) as the first pose. She suggested we then drop over into a backbend, after which we could just kick ourselves back up to Headstand (Sirsasana) and then come down. No preliminary warm-up was offered. "Just do it" was her motto. The first time was fun and easy for me. She suggested we keep going. The second time, as I lifted off the floor from the backbend, hoping to come up easily to Headstand (Sirsasana), I heard an inner crack and felt a searing twinge in my lower lumbar region. I was crestfallen.

Being new to yoga and flexible in my lower back, I was unaware of how to move through the center of my body. I was prone to just whipping my agile spine around. I had caused a vertebral subluxation, or spinal misalignment, which causes interference in the nerve pathways, impeding the transmission of vital information between the cells and the brain. It was a long road to recovery, with many lessons learned in the process. I discovered chiropractors and acupuncturists and found that I needed to build core body strength. I learned the therapeutic style of yoga with Gary Kraftsow and T. K. V. Desikachar, which sent me in another valuable direction. Regrettably I had lost my capacity for advanced backbends, but I was soon able to resume my strong practice without pain.

My back injury inspired me to deepen my investigation of the less popular style of practice called Yin yoga with Paul Grilley. (Yin yoga is a system of long-held, passive floor poses that are similar to but not exactly like restorative postures.) Paul's style at that time was quiet and focused inward. He would come into a pose and we would all follow suit, remaining inward-focused, silent, and motionless until he moved to the next shape, the signal that we could as well. After a few months of this, I began to notice how my lower back seemed to be growing healthier and more comfortable each day. My active flow practice was continuing to develop a core stability in my abdominal and lower back muscles, while the Yin practice seemed to be stimulating the circulation of chi (life force energy) into my deepest spinal region, helping regenerate the fluid content in the joints while increasing the health of my spine.

I loved how I felt after each Yin session, which made me interested in learning more about how these long-held yoga postures influenced not only my flexibility, but my overall health and mental well-being. I had learned about the energy body in yoga but found that by adding some understanding about *meridians* (the term used in Chinese medicine for energy pathways) and organ health, I could broaden and deepen my ability to personalize my practice. It was like having two transparent maps that could be overlaid, providing a much clearer and more distinct picture of my whole inner terrain. When I learned that the balance of the meridian system affects the integrity within and between the body and mind, I became motivated to practice "yin-style" poses not only to increase my physical agility, but to stabilize and replenish my energetic vitality and mental clarity as well.

Although I felt healthier when I practiced regularly, I did not know how specific poses created specific changes. I did not know, for instance, why my often-sensitive, red eyes would clear after doing a seated, wide-leg forward bend. I did not know then that the Liver meridian runs along the inner legs and is connected to the health of the eyes. I just knew I felt better and that was enough—for a while.

Integrating Chinese Medicine with Yoga

As I began to study more about Chinese medicine and some of the basics of Taoism, my yoga practice was enhanced and became more skillful. It was like learning to be my own personal acupuncturist—only without the needles. I learned about the twelve specific meridians that my practice could affect in beneficial ways and how each organ has many energetic components that affect us physically, emotionally, and mentally. I began sequencing my daily practice according to what needed attention. For instance, as I learned about the symptoms of kidney chi disharmonies, I recognized my own imbalances right away. When the kidney chi is not balanced, we may experience

lower back pain, poor circulation in the lower body, or unhealthy reproductive organs.

My back problem was my first clue that I had kidney chi issues, as well as itchiness in my legs from poor circulation whenever I would go for a run, and I've had an ovarian cyst. The deeper I delved into meridian concepts, the more enthusiastic I became about appropriately personalizing my yoga practice. For this reason, I have included in this book the pertinent details about meridian health that I feel can help everyone become more sensitive and skillful in their yoga practice.

You don't have to be a practicing Taoist or an acupuncturist to benefit from the ancient wisdom that the Chinese yogis have accumulated. Just as my brother-in-law, who is a double black belt in tae kwon do, loves how yoga complements his practice, I think yoga practitioners can benefit from understanding relevant aspects of Chinese medicine.

I have become a much healthier person as a result of yoga and holistic therapies, but I am still amazed at how my overall immune system and vitality have changed since I began including Yin yoga in my daily practice. I am so thankful that I now know how to give myself a daily dose of chi balancing. This has diminished the excessive attention (many sessions of acupuncture and chiropractic) my body once needed, allowing me to turn my focus more toward opening and freeing my heart and mind.

Integrating Buddhism with Yoga

During my first ten years of practicing yoga, I was still very unaware and restless. I told myself I was practicing to uncover an alert and spacious yogic heart/mind, but I was really motivated by a desire to feel good physically. I had no understanding of how to train my mind. Not only was my yoga practice affected by this lack of mind training, but my fickle and distracted mind was the source of much of my anguish.

One day, as I found myself looking for yet another book about meditation, I came across a sign in the bookstore that changed my life. On a table was a slogan written in beautiful calligraphy that practically yelled at me, "Meditation, the only way in and the only way out!" I felt as if someone had slapped me. It was time to stop distracting myself with books about meditation and actually take up the practice itself.

Since there were no meditation classes at the yoga studios I was going to (curious thing), I decided to look for a Buddhist group. I had read that unlike most yoga classes, they did not just espouse the benefits of meditation, they actually practiced it, often for seemingly grotesque amounts of time. After about a year of going to weekly Vipassana meditation classes, I felt it was time to really commit. I naively plunged into a ten-day meditation retreat, sitting for more than ten hours a day. I falsely assumed that my ten years of dedicated yoga practice would give me an advantage over others without such a background. Needless to say, it was the greatest challenge of my life to that point, not only for my highly distracted and irritable mind (that much I expected), but for my body as well.

After twenty minutes of trying to sit absolutely still with my legs crossed on a meditation cushion I was in excruciating pain, just as anyone would be. For the first few days I felt imprisoned in my own physical agony and often chastised myself for attending. This dramatic reaction harkened back to my initial distaste for yoga, so I convinced myself that I had better stay the course and give it a chance.

Surprisingly, as the days wore on, I began to notice an increased ability to be with the pains I was feeling (everywhere in my body) without having to move. Even though I was used to holding Yin poses for several minutes, I had never sat this still for hours on end. This capacity for greater and greater physical tolerance, as well as the mental clarity I experienced, had a profound effect on me. As the retreat drew to a close, I felt uncharacteristically open, vulnerable, and grounded inside myself in a way I never had before. I left feeling committed to allowing time each day for meditation in my practice.

After the retreat, I reflected on the Yin practice and how emotionally tense I felt when physical sensations were really strong, especially since I had no tools for how to deal with the pain in my body or the distractions in my mind. Now that I knew how to meditate, I anticipated that my Yin practice would be a place to improve my meditation skills, while my meditation practice would enhance my capacity to stay with my experience in Yin postures.

It was during this time that I started going to a meditation group at the Berkeley Buddhist Monastery once a week. In each session, a talk was given detailing some aspect of the Buddhist path, followed by an hour of sitting practice. After a few weeks, I decided to place myself in the back of the room, out of everyone's view, so I could do some long-held Yin poses while listening to the discourse. I was amazed at how different I felt as a result. Not only was my meditation posture much more comfortable after a few Yin postures than it had ever been, but I discovered that my attention was infinitely more connected to the rhythm of the lecture when I was simultaneously feeling into my body. I felt as though I was receiving the talk not only through the intellectual door of my mind, but also through the pores and cells of my body.

After many weeks, I realized that the dharma talks were seeping into me in a deeply alchemical way. Although I could not remember all I had heard, I was finding an immediacy of application as I attempted to put the teachings into practice then and there in my bodily experience. The Yin poses inevitably triggered emotional and physical challenges, so I began to relate to the strong sensations and my reactions to them with less resistance and more willingness to feel. Since the Yin style of yoga offers an opportunity to cultivate a nondefensive attitude toward sensations, I have found this particular style to be a perfect training ground for learning the Buddhist principles of mindfulness.

As my daily practice expanded to include contemplative aspects, I reflected on the fact that my previous yoga practice had been motivated by a constant desire to change myself. Although this seemed like a healthy interest (and, of course, is in many ways), I began to realize that I was so busy altering the landscape that I often failed to pause and enjoy the view. I was unable to simply value my body (or my life, for that matter) in its current condition, just as it was.

I now see the fundamental necessity of including both Yin and Yang perspectives and practices to reach true maturity. We need time to relax into ourselves unconditionally just as much as we need to nurture and master new abilities. If we are always intent on improving ourselves, we mask and feed our inner demons of self-loathing and unworthiness. As many Buddhist psychologists proclaim, most people conceal a constrictive array of psychological wounds that they are constantly attempting to avoid or manage, which prevents them from ever feeling deeply at ease inside. Even highly functional and seemingly imperturbable adults are often in desperate need of being seen for who they really are, regardless of their accomplishments.

Drawing from philosopher Ken Wilber's concepts about the contrasting importance of both mother love and father love, I see the Yin practices as developing our inner mother love and the Yang practices as fostering healthy father love. Mother love is connected with beingness; father love is aligned with evolution. Mother love lets us value ourselves and others just as we are, whereas father love knows there is always more to learn and room for change. Mother love promotes willing acceptance, while father love develops inspiration toward improvement. A skillful yoga practice can allow both sides of our nature to be inhabited, the receptive, allowing side (yin) and the dynamic, engaging qualities (yang). Ultimately we need both in healthy doses to grow into sane and functional adults who are able to experience authentic intimacy with ourselves and others. When we have divorced these essential attributes, it is like hopping around on one foot—we are easily thrown off balance by the slightest challenge.

The shadow side of imbalanced mother love, or yin excess, expresses itself in our behavior as a collapse of motivation, chronic complacency, feelings of victimization, or apathetic disconnect. This is exemplified in an overly passive woman who cannot take care of herself. On the other hand, an overabundance of father love, or yang influences, encourages restless dissatisfaction and judgmental perfectionism, which pave the road toward intolerant fanaticism. Wherever there is an absence of the feminine yin principle, we see the body—and by extension, the earth—treated as an object, tender emotions denied, and all fragile and vulnerable sides of life aggressively undermined. Yin without yang causes ineptitude, whereas yang without yin can range from cold insensitivity to outright abuse.

Since many of our daily activities are improvement based and yang oriented, our yoga and meditation practices need to have a strong yin element for us to heal this culturally ingrained imbalance. As Buddhist psychiatrist Mark Epstein suggests, the meditative mood is analogous with "an optimal parenting stance," a nonthreatening holding environment that is neither invasive (overly yang) nor abandoning (overly yin).

After many years of integrating my studies in transpersonal psychology, my love of many styles of yoga, and the practices and insights of Buddhism, I now see how each lineage is a transparent map, which when placed on top of the others, widens my ability to chart a course through my inner labyrinth. The various traditions act as guides rather than absolute authorities. In this book, I share my investigation of the synthesis of these spiritual disciplines. I recommend that you read through the whole book first, as this will give you a deeper understanding of how yoga and mindfulness complement each other, after which you can begin the practice sessions of Yin/Yang yoga and mindfulness meditation. My hope is that this book will encourage you to go beyond mere intellectual understanding and that through a commitment to daily inquiry and practice you will discover your inner refuge, the dwelling place of true freedom.

3
Meridian Theory

F OR THOUSANDS OF YEARS, yoga and Chinese medicine have postulated the belief that physical existence is animated by a dynamic energy system that, although unseen, is nonetheless the source or essence of all manifestation. This primordial energy, or chi, is the vital force in all life and is the foundation of all vitality. It is inseparable from movement and change, and it is thought to be what causes the planets to rotate, our brains to think, and our hearts to beat. Not a single blink of the eye or memory in the mind occurs without chi underlying it.

The ancients suggest that this activating energy flows through the body in particular invisible pathways called meridians (Chinese system), or *nadis* (Indian system), like rivers of energy that create a comprehensive network that interconnects and encapsulates the tissues and organs in the human body. These meridians flow through all tissues and bones, moistening the joints and connecting the interior of the body with the exterior. The strength and flow of the meridian system is essential for the harmonious balance in our body and mind. Energy that is weak and lacks vibrancy is called deficient chi, while energy that flows in distorted patterns of movement is called stagnant chi. Healthy chi has the complementary qualities of stable strength and smooth mobility. Committing to a daily, balanced yoga practice is a vital way of enlivening both deficient and stagnant chi disorders (the precursors of all illness) that occur regularly in all of us.

The Meridian theory posited by many masters, such as Dr. Hiroshi Motoyama and his student Paul Grilley, suggests that the connective tissues of the body house a liquid-rich and highly sensitive energy system that can be influenced positively by the way the body is treated. Many practices from various wisdom traditions include a component of chi enhancement disciplines—such as yoga, tai chi, qigong, prostrations, visualizations, mantra, and so on—to enliven the body and mind. If we look at what these diverse styles have in common, we can see a pattern of four specific ways to assist the migration of chi.

The first is a healing modality that incorporates the insertion of needles at particular points on the body along the meridians where chi collects and/or disperses. This method is the basis of the ancient system of acupuncture. It is an extremely complementary addition to a daily yoga practice to help balance the system, particularly when illness or injury has already set in. This healing art offers a strong support to help harmonize whatever within us has lost its equilibrium and needs added assistance to heal. The other three ways can all be accessed through a yoga practice.

The second way to enhance and restore energy is to place the body in particular shapes to both pull on and pressurize tissues. This effort elicits the body's natural repair response, coaxing chi and blood to flood into these sites, making them stronger and better lubricated—literally, more usable in the future. Most forms of exercise, when done regularly and with an appropriate amount of rest afterward, stimulate the circulation in the whole body. There is an added benefit of practicing movements that stem from the wisdom traditions rather than conventional exercise: the complementary emphasis on training the mind. Working on the level of the body while simultaneously training the mind deepens our overall sense of well-being in a way that can last beyond the exercise sessions themselves. The last two ways of influencing chi flow involve this level of mind training.

The third way to mobilize the energy within is to lengthen and deepen the breath. Yogis have found that by controlling the breath (a practice called *pranayama*), we oxygenate the blood while increasing the flow of prana into more harmonious patterns of distribution. This practice has a calming and clarifying effect on the emotions and mind, and it is possible to practice while doing yoga poses, particularly in a Yin practice. A number of different methods will be discussed in later chapters.

The fourth way to stimulate chi is the most direct and often the most difficult method. It relates to the focus of mind we bring to our movements. Yogis and scientists agree that our state of mind is directly related to the quality of our energy body. Someone with a distracted mind will have scattered and destabilized chi flow, whereas someone with a focused mind will have smooth, even-flowing prana. Yogis discovered long ago that prana flows where our attention goes. Our mental focus can collect and enhance our energy for healing purposes, as well as for the function of expanding consciousness beyond the mundane realms. Someone who has a focused mind that is free of emotional afflictions will experience very few chi disharmonies. It is a focused

and spacious mind that draws chi toward the core of the body like a magnet. When our energy rests along the center of our body, we no longer experience the distraction of fragmented energetic and emotional dissonances, allowing us to move more easily into contemplative investigations in meditation. With maturity, meditative concentration blossoms into nondual awareness, a nondistracted yet spacious alertness that recognizes the inseparability of emptiness and form.

A balanced yoga practice can potentially comprise the last three methods of chi enhancement: doing postures to stimulate the muscles, blood, and meridians housed in the connective tissues; engaging in conscious, slow breathing to regulate the nervous system and amplify the quality of energy; and focusing the mind while disentangling consciousness from distractions.

The Basics of Taoism

It is only by Qi that the planets move, the sun shines, the wind blows, the elements exist, and human beings live and breathe. It is the cohesion of the bodymindspirit and the integration of the myriad aspects of each individual human being. It is spoken of with reverence because it is the basis of life and when gone awry, the basis of disease.

—Dianne M. Connelly, *Traditional Acupuncture*

In Taoism, the essential essence of all life is called *wu chi*. It is translated as the Infinite, the Great Void, or sometimes the stillness within movement. It is synonymous with the terms Brahman in Hinduism (the totality of the universe) and Sunyata in Buddhism, referring to the unqualifiable intelligent vastness. This is the formless dimension that nourishes spirit and is the essence of chi within every living thing. It is the limitless, all-pervading force underlying all existence.

Chi

Everything in the universe, organic and inorganic is composed of and defined by its Qi. Chinese thought does not easily distinguish between matter and energy, but we can think of chi as matter on the verge of becoming energy and energy at the point of Materializing.

—TED KAPTCHUCK,
The Web That Has No Weaver

The power of the Infinite, or wu chi, stepped down into the everyday world is simply called chi (pronounced "chee"). It is sometimes seen as *Ki* or *Qi* in Japanese, linking the concept of energy with the mental capacity of intention, indicating that the mind has a major influence on how chi functions. It represents the Infinite in a condensed form. *Chi* is the Chinese equivalent of the Sanskrit term *prana,* or *lung* in Tibetan. It is the link between the spirit, the mind, and the body. It is the foundation of all life, the vital force behind all of creation.

Chi is often translated into English as "energy," "breath," "air," "vital essence," or "the activating energy of the universe." It is neither created nor destroyed and is constantly transforming itself to reappear in different ways. These wisdom traditions believe that all states of existence are temporary manifestations of chi, which is the animating factor of all living beings.

Chi is emitted and absorbed by every living thing. Yogis and Taoists discovered long ago that opening the major energy channels (meridians) increases the circulation of chi and amplifies our energy, enhancing our capacity to absorb more chi. It is within us and all around us. Trees, for example, give off different chi essences. I remember Master Motoyama suggesting that we find the kind of trees we love to be near and sit under them regularly, as the chi they emit can help balance our own internal chi. He also said that the reason we sometimes feel really good in the presence of some people and not others is because the chi the former send out matches our chi on the inside. Something similar holds true for strange feelings of unease we may have with certain people, even when we have never spoken with them. The chi they emit does not intermingle well with our energy.

Yin and Yang

Taoist yogis suggest that as chi condenses into the physical realm, it splits into two complementary polarities called yin and yang. Chi is constantly configuring and dispersing in alternating cycles, endlessly materializing in different ways. These two energies are of the same essence (they are both chi) but reflect different qualities of energy and are ultimately inseparable. They can be understood as the positive and negative poles of existence that are intrinsic to all creation.

Taoists use the famous black-and-white circle to represent this energetic play in physical reality. The black side represents chi's yin aspects and refers to those elements that are darker, harder to see, or more deeply hidden. It is often likened to the shady side of a mountain. The white side represents the yang aspects of energy. It is the brighter, more obvious, surface part of reality. It is the sunny side of the mountain. They are shown in a circle, the representation of life's cyclical nature and inherent unity. Although they appear as separate, polar opposites, the line drawn between them is not a straight one. It is curved in an S shape, representing the eternal intertwinement of these two coessential essences. They are like two rivers constantly meeting, one side continually changing into and becoming the other. There is never one without the other, as the

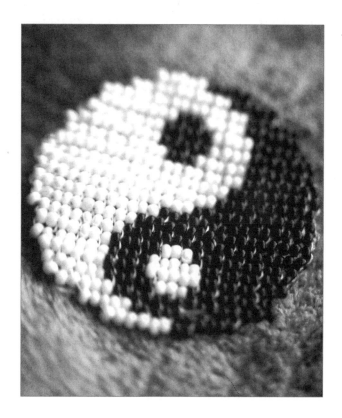

opposite-color dot in each side depicts. All states of existence are temporary manifestations of a blend of yin and yang chi.

Similarly, the yogic term for any physical-based practice, *hatha,* reflects these two distinct yet unified energies. *Hatha* can be broken into its two parts: *ha,* meaning the warming, sunlike manifestations (from the sun god Surya); and *tha,* meaning the cooling or moon elements (from the moon goddess Chandra). Hatha yoga is a marriage of ha and tha, a balanced equilibrium of yin and yang energies. The terms *yin* and *yang* reflect these same coessential opposites.

When we refer to something as yin, we mean that it is cooler, less mobile, more hidden, or in the center, feminine, and closer to the earth. Conversely, things that are yang are warmer, more pliant, superficial, masculine, and closer to the heavens. These terms are relational, meaning they are not separate, static truths existing in a vacuum. As they emerge out of the same source, one or the other is simply more dominant at different times, yet they remain in a constant dialogue with each other, seeking a natural equilibrium with their opposite energy.

Yin and *yang* are adjectives that describe the way chi manifests and are often used in a comparative way. In terms of the human body, the lower half is closer to the ground, which makes it the yin half, compared to the upper body, which is closer to the sky, making it more yang. The inner body is closer to the center or hidden, so it is considered yin to the yang outer layers. The bones and connective tissues that bind them (ligaments) are closer to the inner body and therefore can be described as yin tissues as opposed to the skin, muscles, and fascia, which can be called yang tissues.

Using this yin/yang analogy, any physical practice that involves rhythmic movement and engages muscles can be considered a Yang practice, even though some styles are certainly more yang in nature than others. Yang yoga practices primarily target strengthening and lengthening muscles, which of course also improves the health of the organs and bones as well as the circulatory and respiratory systems. This includes all kinds of Hatha yoga styles, including Iyengar, Ashtanga, Anusara, and Bikram, as well as other activities like running, biking, swimming, or hiking. (Note that these practices often contain yin aspects as well.) Yin tissues are affected during a Yang practice, but the emphasis on muscle engagement and movement and the shorter duration of the poses predominantly (but not exclusively) attracts the distribution of chi into the yang tissues, while enlivening the energetic, responsive characteristics of mind.

Conversely, a practice that is mainly stationary and allows many of the muscle groups to soften, while exposing the joints to pressure as the skeleton is pulled apart, can be considered a Yin practice. Yang tissues are also stretched and influenced in Yin yoga, but the longer the body is still, the more the chi becomes concentrated in the deeper yin tissues (the bones and ligaments). As we settle into the stillness, our yin aspects of being—our contemplative, receptive qualities—are also enhanced. Depending on whether we want to have a greater effect on the inner or outer parts of the body, or our capacity to surrender or become active, we will practice yoga postures in a consciously different manner. Neither way is better, and ideally we learn to be skillful in both, allowing these complementary practices to enhance our capacity for body-mind vitality and integrity.

When we want to target yin tissues to maintain their healthy capacity, we need to understand that they cannot be enhanced in the same way as our muscles, or yang tissues. Yin tissues, being naturally less elastic with much less fluid content than yang tissues, do not have the same ability to stretch and elongate. Yin tissues need to be pulled and compressed gently in order to maintain their pliancy within their natural ranges of motion, as well as to nourish the meridians coursing through them.

To maintain or relubricate healthy yin tissues, we need to ask more of them *appropriately.* We need to do our yoga poses in a yin way. This means that instead of coming into a pose for a short amount of time and hugging the bones close together by engaging our muscles (a skillful way to work with yang tissue), we have to pull the skeleton apart nonaggressively and with appropriate pressure and then remain stationary a while, allowing the muscles to remain stretched but without engaging them. Since ligaments do not have a high fluid content, they do not respond to use as rapidly as yang tissues. So instead of staying in a pose for many breaths, in Yin yoga, we stay in them for many minutes.

Whereas a Yang practice bears some similarity to physical therapy, the Yin practice of steady stress is similar to the healing modality of traction. The skeleton is slowly pulled apart in a tensile stretch and held in place for longer periods. Each session of three- to five-minute holds or more is not an attempt to *stretch* the ligaments but to *load* them appropriately, thereby initiating the body's natural response to stress by stimulating the circulation of chi through them.

If we stress the ligaments appropriately in a nonaggressive way, they literally grow back a little bit stronger and more pliant after each session. Over time, with consistent practice, we can maintain elasticity in the joints throughout our lives. A very skillfull practitioner can even help stimulate the healing of degenerative tissues in areas that are already compromised, as it is chi that heals.

For instance, we can practice Cobra Pose (Bhujangasana) with arms bent, back muscles engaged, and legs active; stay in it for only a few breaths; and repeat it a few times. This makes it a Yang practice because it targets the increase of chi into the musculature that helps the body bend up and back. The chi distribution is emphasized in the muscles along the spine and movement of blood into the back of the body, as well as the arms and legs.

Conversely, we can take the same pose, straighten our arms and rest in them for support, relax many of the muscle groups in our back, and allow our legs to be passive. This would classify as a Yin practice—this time called Seal Pose (see page 43), amplifying the flow of chi into the connective tissues along the spine (the longitudinal ligaments) and increasing the chi distribution into the energy channels that flow through these tissues (where the Kidney meridian is). We can also choose to do this pose with some of the muscles relaxed and some engaged, depending on the amount of sensation that is appropriate for us in our spine. How much to activate and how much to relax in any given pose is the responsibility of each practitioner to discern and can only come from subjective experience.

Like Cobra Pose (Bhujangasana), many yoga postures can be broken down into a Yin or Yang way of practice, changing the target area of chi distribution from the less elastic core tissues and bones in the Yin approach to the more mobile, superficial tissues or muscles in the Yang. This allows a high degree of creativity in how we incorporate both styles. Some people find it beneficial to emphasize all Yin postures one day and then move through the active Yang sequences the following day. Less flexible people often prefer to start with Yang sequences, then slow down into a Yin style toward the end of a session. Those with more bendy bodies might prefer to start with some Yin poses (to prevent their muscles from taking the bulk of the stretch when they are warmed up) and then move on to the Yang postures. Still others do some Yang poses in the morning to get their energy moving and then do a Yin session in the evening to unwind after a long day. These are all viable options that elicit various effects. (See the appendix for sequencing suggestions.) The important point is learning how to gauge ourselves appropriately, to notice any imbalances, and to skillfully apply a practice that helps the body-mind's natural inclination toward equilibrium.

As we create time for ourselves to practice more regularly, we begin to identify our moods and overall personalities as being either more introverted (yin) or outgoing (yang). Creating a practice that encourages the opposite side of our nature is a direct way to increase our overall well-being, as well as to help to expand our psychological maturity. We can still include the parts of the practice that we easily gravitate toward (a quiet practice when we feel contemplative or a vigorous session when we feel exuberant), but we do it with a renewed recognition that balance will elude us if we only address one side of our nature while excluding its complement.

A fast-moving, fast-talking stockbroker may love the pace of Ashtanga yoga or the heat and endurance required for Bikram yoga. Such practices may serve this kind of person well, but if he is not aware of the habit of speed and distraction he has collected, he will not develop the sensitivity necessary to yield and reflect, open and listen, which are essential qualities of his yin nature. As a result, aggression and ambition in his practice (and life) will go unnoticed, fueling the habit of striving. Although this attitude prevails in competitive sports, when we strain to produce a desired result in yoga, it leads us away from inner peace and insight, instead creating more grasping, a risk of injury, and increased egocentrism.

Another kind of person may be naturally quiet and introverted, or self-protective, tentative, and passive. Although a Yin practice may come naturally, she will also benefit from including a regular Yang practice. She will need to build strength and endurance, allowing these yang features of her nature to emerge and grow. She may need to emphasize developing a healthy will by making active commitments and following through with them. When doing a Yin practice, she will benefit from heightening her alert attention to body sensations to prevent disconnecting from her moments by spacing out and "hanging out" in the protective cocoon of a passive practice. I have found that most people usually need both kinds of practices to ensure their overall well-being and integrity, even though one or the other style of practice may be given more emphasis to help balance them at different junctures of their lives.

Whatever our psychological propensity may be, a balanced yoga practice allows us to become increasingly sensitive to the changing rhythms of our lives. Some days we may feel extremely fatigued or emotionally drained. On these days we can benefit from lots of Yin yoga, some gentle pranayama, and meditation to restore and replenish us. Other days the imbalance may stem from an excess of activity and overmanagement of many details. This causes a constant drain on our chi account and can pull us into an addiction to constantly overworking. A mindful Yang practice that is closely linked with the breath and focus of the mind can help redirect this inner chaos. We want to refresh and enliven our energy through movement, but we also need to include a Yin practice and meditation to begin to influence the more receptive, intuitive side. This can help us develop patience and tolerance for slower rhythms, as well as leading us to deeper discoveries about ourselves.

Although both styles of practice are essential, it is often easier for most people to learn a Yang practice before a Yin one and to learn asanas (poses) before they endeavor to meditate. Even in perfectly healthy adults with moderate mobility, the need to be still for an extended period brings up not only difficult sensations, but chaotic and often intolerable thoughts and feelings as well. After the body has rested from physical activity, the muscles revert back to their average amount of fluid content. The physical discomfort a person—even someone who is quite agile—may feel in a lengthy floor pose or meditation is often not located in the hamstrings or back muscles. It arises predominantly in the knees, hips, sacral area, and lumbar spine, which are all joint sites, or yin tissues.

Although the challenge of being still seems to stem from physical discomfort, for most people, it is predominantly a mental issue. Learning to open to difficulty without resistance is the domain of mindfulness training and is a highly practical and liberating tool for life. The Yin poses (more so than the Yang) can be a viable way to begin a meditation practice, helping us slowly become more comfortable in our bodies and minds. After learning how to be still for these short but potent three- to five-minute intervals, a meditation practice of ten to twenty minutes does not seem so daunting.

The process of learning to sense which combination of poses in which sequence will best help replenish and enliven the body, heart, and mind is both the burden and the privilege of each practitioner. Teachers and teachings are essential to begin this process and to continually upgrade our choices once we are on our way, but no one can live inside our own unique experience and determine for us how best to practice and live. That has to come from our own trial and error, continually fueled and renewed by a deep interest in personal freedom through self-discovery.

Yin/Yang Organs

All substances can be described as either yin or yang, depending on their primary function and their relationship to something else. For example, if our discussion is about physical activities, any form of yoga would be more of a yin choice than other sports, because the focus and intention in yoga is more introspective. If the discussion changes to the different styles of yoga, then doing a sequence of standing poses and inversions would be more of a yang choice than doing long-held forward bends.

When we speak about the body itself, the organs and bones are nearer the core and therefore could be considered more yin, while the muscles and skin are nearer the surface, making them more yang. If we are speaking about the organs in relation to each other, they can be characterized as either yin or yang also, yet every organ has both a supportive, nourishing yin element and an active yang element. Yin organs are those concerned with the pure energy of fundamental substances such as chi, blood, essence (*jing*), and spirit (*shen*). They transform, regulate, and store these primary energies. The yin organs are the kidneys, liver, spleen, heart, and lungs.

Yang organs are involved with impure substances such as undigested food, urine, and waste. Their job is to receive and digest food, absorbing useful components, while transmitting or excreting waste. The yang organs are the urinary bladder, gallbladder, stomach, and small and large intestines.

The Five-Element Theory

As we learn about the energy-related functions of the organs and meridians (and how to balance them in our yoga practice), it is helpful to think of them as operating in similar ways to substances in nature. The ancient Taoists studied nature to determine what universal principles could be applied to humans' health and well-being.

The five elements in nature are drawn from fire, water, wood, metal, and earth. These five were chosen based on the observations of ancient Asian philosophers who theorized that the natural world as well as the human body incorporated each of these elemental characteristics. Chinese medicine uses a time-tested, diagnostic model based on this theory to analyze how the various parts of a person's body and mind interact to affect health. These five elements symbolically express the physical elements as five processes of energy. They are not literal designations but can be thought of as approximations of behavior.

The five natural elements are matched up with the five yin organs and represent how each yin/yang pair behaves on an energetic level when in or out of balance. The heart and small intestine act most like fire, or energy that rises. When their energy is depleted, we feel cold-hearted or depressed; when there is an excess, we feel aggressive and fiery. Of the other four pairs, water (likened to energy sinking) is associated with the kidneys and urinary bladder; wood (energy expanding) is linked with the liver and gallbladder; metal (the regulation and communication of energy) is related to the lungs and large intestine; and earth (stable or centered energy) describes the spleen and stomach. As with the universe at large, every aspect of human beings, including the mind, emotions, and physical substances can be associated with the relationship between the five elements. The table on page 20 classifies the many components and how they relate to each element.

Two Internal Sources of Chi

According to Chinese yogis, two main internal sources of chi constantly influence the human body. These sources consist of prenatal, or hereditary energy, which is with us from conception until death; and acquired chi, which is all energy developed after birth—absorbed from food (grain chi) and from breathing air (natural air chi).

Prenatal energy refers to our inherited constitution. This energy is nourished in the womb and comprises our genetic codes intertwined with our karma (accumulated energetic seeds bound by current intentions and reactions). This is the storehouse of energy we are working with from birth until death. Prenatal chi is a given and will not change dramatically once our physical life is set in motion, although it can be depleted or enhanced depending on our life experiences and choices. This is the main reason why we need to personalize our yoga practice to best suit our constitution's daily needs. Prenatal chi is stored in the kidneys.

	WOOD	FIRE	EARTH	METAL	WATER
Yin organ	Liver	Heart	Spleen	Lungs	Kidneys
Yang organ	Gallbladder	Small intestine	Stomach	Large intestine	Urinary bladder
Tissue	Tendon Muscle	Blood vessels	Blood Muscle	Skin	Bones Teeth Joint lubrication
Controls	Flow of chi Inner disposition Detoxification	Circulation Assimilation	Digestion Distribution	Respiration Elimination	Reproductive organs Lower back health Urinary system Blood purification Energetic vitality
Chakra	Manipura	Anahata	Manipura	Vishuddhi	Muladhara Svadhisthana
Sense organ	Eyes	Tongue	Mouth	Nose	Ear
Liquid emitted	Tears	Sweat	Saliva	Mucus	Urine
Natural cycle	Birth	Growth	Maturity	Harvest	Store
Nourishes	Nails	Complexion	Lips	Body hair	Head hair
Emotions	Anger Compassion	Hate Love	Anxiety Equanimity	Sorrow Courage	Fear Wisdom
Color	Green	Red	Yellow	White	Blue/black
Season	Spring	Summer	Indian Summer	Fall	Winter
Climate	Windy	Hot	Damp	Dry	Cold
Taste	Sour	Bitter	Sweet	Spicy	Salty

Kidney jing, as it is called, refers to our unique constitution (see chapter 6 for more detail).

All other acquired internal sources have a direct influence on our kidney jing. Grain chi is derived from the digestion of foods and liquids and acts to either enhance or reduce energy, depending on whether the chi of the food is in harmony with our constitution or not. Some foods help heal the system's imbalances; some are considered neither harmful nor helpful (neutral); and others act as poisons, causing our system to go into overload to properly digest and discard their harmful components. Understanding our particular makeup is of vital importance in taking care of ourselves properly, as many seemingly innocuous or even healing foods can act as poisons to some people's systems. Ayurveda and Chinese medicine have created an elaborate healing science by understanding different individuals' needs. (See the Suggested Readings in the back of this book to explore this aspect further.)

Another internal source is called natural air chi, and it is absorbed through our lungs from the air we breathe. It is absolutely necessary for us to have access to fresh air that is free of polluting toxins for our bodies and minds to function properly. This is becoming an increasingly rare commodity in our environmentally overloaded atmospheres, which has severe repercussions for all living beings. Practicing yoga and pranayama outside or in rooms well ventilated with fresh air is essential for overall health. Regularly taking walks in nature is as vitally important for well-being as are daily internal practices.

Chi Functions and Dysfunctions

Although formless, chi is perceived according to its specific functions. All normal chi has a number of functions that are responsible for all the physical and energetic integrity in the body-mind organism. These functions include movement, protecting the body from harmful environmental elements, extracting energy from the food we eat, keeping substances like blood in their appropriate pathways, and maintaining an adjustable yet balanced body temperature.

Although the same chi flows through the spleen as through the kidneys, each organ is thought to have its own chi, because the activity within the organs is different. And just as there are specifics within organ chi, organ chi is thought to be distinct from meridian chi, which also has variations within it. Meridian chi flows along the many subtle pathways, linking the various organs and tissues, and yet, Kidney meridian chi has different features from Liver meridian chi, for example.

Healthy chi is described as being both strong and mobile. When its quality of strength is impaired, it is considered a yin condition (deficient chi). This refers to underactivity and a pattern of disharmony in the flow of chi. Deficient chi develops whenever chi is unable to perform one of its essential functions. Examples of deficient chi include chronic lethargy and frequent sickness.

When the mobility of our chi is impaired, it is considered a yang condition (stagnant chi). This is associated with both incongruous or unrestrained movements of chi, or a sluggish flow of chi that may be rough or discordant in some way. Like water that collects and putrefies in a pond, stagnant blockages of chi underlie most illnesses and ailments.

Healthy chi has a particular quality and fluidity of energy; it is able to nourish and balance the functions of all the organs and systems synchronistically. This balancing is called homeostasis, which is the maintenance of constancy in the internal environment. Yin yoga can be considered both preventive and restorative. The meditative practice of remaining still for long periods without an agenda of manipulation influences and enhances the yin aspects (quality) of chi, while tugging on the connective tissues affects the redistribution of chi, enhancing its yang aspect (mobility). When we practice Yin yoga, we enrich the quality of chi by slowing down and surrendering to our experience. This unhurried and unambitious attitude combined with the ability to feel deeply attentive to our bodies diminishes our stress levels and allows our system to discharge excess tensions that have built up through unaware living as well as past frozen traumas that are locked in our tissues. As we settle down and drop into mindfulness, this discharge from our energy body is naturally calming and balancing, enhancing the overall quality of chi. Activating chi distribution in the tissues through pressure or appropriate stress, as in each pose of both Yin and Yang practices, stimulates the mobilization of chi throughout the various meridians and organs, thereby enhancing its fluidity. I have found the Yin practice in particular to enhance both fundamental functions of healthy chi—its strong quality and its fluid mobility.

4

Beginning a Yin/Yang Yoga Practice

THERE ARE TWO INSPIRING MOTIVATIONS to practice yoga regularly. The first is that daily inward-drawn attention teaches us how to heal and fully inhabit ourselves, developing an attitude of attentiveness and kindness within us. Patterns of neglect and self-abuse manifest in a myriad of habitual ways. When we regularly turn our attention toward our inner landscape in a yoga practice, we learn how to avoid becoming ensnared by these familiar behaviors. Developing the mind to become our ally rather than a battle zone is one of the most challenging yet rewarding dimensions of our practice. Learning how to live in our bodies in a wholesome way and to be better friends to ourselves becomes the foundation of a compassionate worldview and is a prerequisite for more advanced practices.

The second motivation to take up a daily practice is to accelerate our ability to help, heal, and naturally love others. As our inward practices begin to take root, they rejuvenate our depleted vitality, freeing us from our tensions and reactive habits day by day. Inevitably this helps us become more able to sustain inspired support for and intimacy with others, without disconnecting from self-awareness. Adding practices of loving-kindness (*metta*) and compassion (*karuna*) to our meditation time will help deepen our responsiveness, especially toward those in need or suffering (see page 176 for more information on these practices).

As we begin a Yin/Yang yoga practice, it is helpful to remember that Yin yoga activity is slow, steady, and often stationary, with a sense of core softness and surrender. Yang yoga activity is mobile, builds to an apex before calming down, and maintains a core strength that requires appropriate effort. Just as the black dot in the white side and the white dot in the black side of the Taoist circle remind us that there is no such thing as a purely yin or purely yang reality, every balanced yin activity involves some yang elements and vice versa. The main difference between these different styles of engagement is a matter of degrees—a shift not so much in which poses we choose (for a yoga pose is not in and of itself Yin or Yang) but in how we practice determines whether we target the yin or yang tissues more directly or indirectly.

I remember Paul Grilley describing this yin/yang concept using examples from Taoism. The Chinese yogis believe the yin/yang dynamic in the human body is an unavoidable trajectory from infancy to old age. They describe our early years as our yang phase. We are born into a very soft, pliant body with an excess of moisture in our tissues and a minimum of rigidity. We cannot even hold our heads up for the first few months of life. As we mature, we take on more yin, earth elements of stability. Our bones become firmer, and within a year or so we are able to stand and hold ourselves upright without assistance. Gradually, our yang mobility is balanced with our yin stability, bringing us into our physical prime in our late teens to late twenties.

It is in this decade that we may become star athletes, dancers, or gymnasts—a time when yin/yang equilibrium matched with training and passion can render extreme physical prowess. Most professional competitors have only this brief window of performance ability, although their skill and dedication may improve with age. What is unavoidably their demise is not something their training can help them avert. The difference between an athlete who is eighteen versus one who is thirty-eight is not skill, but ability. The older person has moved into what can be called a yin phase, the aging process. Our tissues naturally begin drying up from our early thirties on. Synovial fluid in our joints (which has an egglike consistency and acts as a joint lubricant) begins to lose its viscosity, causing the physical grace we once may have had to decrease; our movements become less and less smooth, with the risk of injury and the time it takes to heal gradually increasing. This process continues until death, at which time we become completely yin (in rigor mortis).

When we consider the injuries most competent athletes sustain that can cause them to lose their capacity to compete, the problems are often in the knees or hips or along the spine or shoulders. In other words, they harm their joints. These damaged joints inhibit the natural flow of chi within their bodies, not only diminishing their range of motion, which ends their athletic careers, but greatly compromising their organs and overall health as well. For yogis as well as athletes, maintaining and rehabilitating these areas is essential for general well-being, yet joints cannot be enhanced in the same way as muscle tissue can.

Muscles respond well to rhythmic movement because this easily increases their fluid content, giving them more agility and strength. The alternation of contracting and releasing muscles, combined with adequate rest, stimulates the body's natural repair response. This built-in biological rescue remedy occurs when any of our tissues have been used. The body naturally responds by sending an increased blood supply that carries nutrients to the stressed area. From a Meridian theory perspective, this action is the result of stimulating yang chi, which moves the blood and causes the area to become thicker, more mobile, easier to use.

There is little dispute that for healthy circulation, respiration, digestion, and evacuation, we need to regularly move our body in a yang way by engaging the muscles. The risk involved in any physical activity is that the joints do not respond to movement in the same way as the muscles. They are not as elastic because they do not have a high fluid content. Muscles start out at about 75 percent fluid and go up to about 90 percent with vigorous exercise, whereas ligaments are mostly composed of dense fibrous tissue with only about 6 percent fluid content. This is why any good yoga class teaches adequate anatomical understanding to ensure a safe practice.

To protect the joints when we are doing active yoga poses, we need to learn how to move the appropriate core muscles without straining or losing our connection to deep breathing. It is the muscles' job, when engaged properly, to hold the bones closer together. As we bend back and lunge forward, we don't simply thrash our bodies around, compressing and tensing joints in and out of different shapes. Instead, we move with our attention firmly yet buoyantly hugging the midline muscles of the body together; this includes the adductors (inner thigh muscles) in the legs, the erector spinea (along the spine), trapezius (upper shoulder) muscles in the back, and the biceps and deltoids in the upper arms. With proper structural/muscular alignment, our movements will not be aggressive or risky as long as we are within our joints' natural range of motion. This way of practicing yoga is a yang activity done in a safe and healthy way. For this discussion, all practices that involve rhythmic movement and engage muscles will be considered Yang practices.

As mentioned before, as we age, our natural range of motion lessens due to the decrease in all forms of moisture in the body, particularly the synovial fluid in the joint capsules. This is why Yin yoga is a complementary discipline to a Yang practice. It helps prevent joint rigidity and immobility, while also helping to enliven degenerative tissues and simultaneously nourishing the meridians.

Maintaining healthy joint stability is a chief concern for everyone, and as already discussed, learning how to protect our joints as we move around is essential. But joint mobility is also a necessity for a healthy body, especially when considering the implications of the Meridian theory. When a joint hardens through injury or lack of use in its full range of motion, the connective tissues literally shrink-wrap around it, making occasional attempts to expand the range of that joint ever more painful and limited. This reduced pliancy in the joints becomes the main roadblock or traffic jam within the internal chi highways. Constant interruptions of the natural fluidity of chi through the ligaments and bones cause a chain reaction, disturbing both the health of the skeleton and organs, which this yin chi feeds, and creating psychological imbalances as well. (Later chapters discuss each organ's functions.)

Three Main Principles in Yin Postures

There are three main tenets that help nourish the joints in a yoga pose. The first is to come into the chosen shape to an appropriate edge. This means coming into poses nonaggressively and sensitively, allowing the breath to remain slow and unlabored so we can detect the appropriate depth of sensation that we feel we can tolerate. If we attempt to take on too much intensity too soon, our inner state—or mood of resistance—will actually hinder the chi flow, causing more energetic disruptions. If, on the other hand, we do not exert enough tension, avoiding any strong sensations,

we do not allow these areas to expand into their full ranges of motion and it is the pulling and pressure that excites the chi flow into them.

If we are working on an area that is fragile, injured, or hypermobile, we need to do two things. First, we should merely suggest the shape, coming into the pose just enough to stimulate chi flow without any feeling of strain. Second, we need to remain highly focused on the sensations promoted by the pose, thereby refining our meditative attention, while relaxing the rigidity around the painful joint. Of course, we may also need to use props; allowing for modifications and variations to support damaged or destabilized areas. These adjustments are greatly enhanced by the assistance of a skilled teacher in the beginning, but they are also shown in many of the pose variations in this book.

The second tenet to help nourish the joints is to become still and muscularly soft, allowing gravity to have us. Whenever we move, the chi flows more predominantly in the muscles and fasciae. During a Yin practice, we intend to pool chi in the bones and joints, which requires that we diminish movement and settle into the pose. Of course, there will be times when we feel our tissues moistening and naturally drop deeper into a pose. At other times, we may concede that we have gone too far too soon and need to back off. These kinds of adjustments are certainly appropriate. We may also feel our legs falling asleep at times and want to come out to massage the area and bring it back to life before returning to the pose.

The lengthy postural steadiness allows us to develop yin qualities of surrender and observance, a willingness to feel a greater tolerance for uncomfortable experiences. After doing many Yin poses strung together, I have found that a feeling commonly develops that is similar to the effect of a long acupuncture session. My body begins to feel very relaxed and at ease, while my mind feels a heightened sense of clarity and restfulness. My acupuncturist liked to call this "acubliss."

The third tenet is to hold each pose for a while so as to fully nourish the meridians. As with acupuncture, where the acupuncturist does not put the needles in only to take them right back out, we want to coax the chi into particular pathways, help-ing to engorge the respective organs with refined energy. This takes some time and patience. I like to set a timer so that I can let go of wondering how long it has been, freeing my mind to connect to the present moment more easily. For brand-new beginners to this practice, I suggest one to three minutes in each pose, although five minutes is what I teach and practice most often. I find that it is just becoming challenging for people at three minutes, and the extra two-minute intensity can be a wonderful training ground for cultivating a broader capacity to stay with unpleasant sensa-tions (as long as it does not feel risky).

Once we understand why and how to set up a pose and have chosen one to settle into, our first anchor of attention can become the breath in the center of our body. I find that a slow Ujjayi breath allows the mind to drop into quietude best, while also assisting the energetic equilibrium (see page 102). Pranayama is a direct way to influence the distribution of chi and can be practiced formally sometimes during the Yin poses in a very effec-tive way. (I will discuss this in more detail in the next section.)

The steady breath rhythm acts as a barometer for how skillfully we are practicing, and if we pay careful attention, it allows us to refine our ability to detect any tendency toward overaggres-sion or pushing our body too far. When the soft sound, which is similar to waves building under the ocean floor, becomes jagged, forced, or inter-rupted, it is time to back off from the physical in-tensity in order to reconnect with the inner waves of breath flow.

Once we are aligned with our unhindered breath rhythms, we can settle deeper into our ob-serving nature. Since the poses themselves do not require constant thought, we can turn our atten-tion to the subtler aspects of experience.

Attention to the Breath in Yoga Poses

Yogis (and more recently scientists) have discov-ered that prana flows in certain universal patterns that represent our states of consciousness. Con-ventionally, the upper body energy, or wind (vayu), is connected to the inhalation, which convention-ally flows up and out. This is called *prana,* which is not the same as Prana, meaning overall vital en-ergy. Taoists refer to this upper wind as heart en-ergy and likened it to the element of fire, which is upward flowing. Conversely, the lower body wind is linked to the exhalation; it has a tendency to flow down and out and is called *apana,* or kidney energy, which, like water, flows downward. Both Indian and Chinese yogis practice a breathing art intended to bring these polar opposite inner winds toward the center of the body and each other. This practice gathers energy into the central canal, called the *sushumna* (Indian), *uma* (Tibetan), *chong mai* or *du mai* (approximate Taoist concepts), or the "thrusting channel." When the two main aspects of breath collide and intermingle in our core, our consciousness opens into its natural con-templative state, creating an inner atmosphere in which insight and wisdom can percolate.

To influence the way prana flows within us, we have to link our attention to our breath, which is the main catalyst for inner circulation. Remember that *Prana flows where our attention goes.* This be-comes a natural focal point for our attention while surrendering into the long Yin poses, as well as something we can attend to in our Yang practice. Having gathered our attention on a smooth Ujjayi breath (see page 102) that lasts around five seconds for an inhalation and five seconds for an exhalation, we can then focus not only on the breath's length and depth, but also on its direction. As we inhale, we draw our attention from our chest, where we first feel the in-breath, to our pelvic floor, using our attention to encourage the flow from top to bottom. As we exhale, we reverse this pattern and flow from the perineum back up to the heart center.

As we continue to breathe in this way, the upper and lower winds begin to bleed into each other, amplifying the benefits of the inhalation energy when we exhale and enhancing the exha-lation's influence while we inhale. After a while, we can simply rest our attention behind our navel center (the intersection between the chest and the pelvic floor) for longer and longer periods. This area is the power center in the body and is the seat of awareness, called Prana-mind. When we are balanced, we will experience a sense of ease and space in this region. When we are contracted in this region, we block our internal source of power. Negative emotions, stress, and tension accumulate in the belly center. We can begin to untether and release these stagnating patterns when we abide softly in this region, both during our practice and throughout the day.

This collection of breath in the central channel and belly center acts as a resource pool from which to draw refined energy. With this increased energy infusion in our core, we create a reservoir of balanced energy that we can direct into the various regions of the body where it is needed.

5

Organ Health in Yin Yoga

THE HEALTH OF OUR ORGANS is vital to our overall well-being. If we understand their importance on the physical, energetic, and psychological levels, we will be much more motivated to develop a yoga practice that nourishes, protects, and even helps to heal the visceral organs. If we begin to understand our own constitution and its potential weaknesses, we can learn to sequence postures that best enable our body to maintain its equilibrium.

In Chinese medicine, the function of the organs is not measured solely by the anatomical roles they play, but by their energetic constitutions as well. Even though the organs work as a matrix of interdependent influences, each has a physical, an energetic, and an emotional function that directly contributes to psychosomatic health.

The organs in Chinese medicine are inextricably linked to the health of the meridians that flow through them. Each yin organ and meridian has a direct sister-brother relationship with a complementary yang organ and meridian. This means that what we do to one immediately affects the other. Although the pairs of yin/yang organs have different anatomical functions, their energetic, emotional, and mental qualities are so intimately intertwined that I have simply categorized these distinctions in the description of each yin organ, while giving a brief anatomical description of the complementary yang organ.

There are fourteen major meridians, twelve of which are considered regular and can be positively affected by doing yoga poses. These twelve yin and yang meridians are specifically connected to six yin-yang pairs of organs. The kidneys (yin) are paired with the urinary bladder (yang), the liver (yin) with the gallbladder (yang), the spleen (yin) with the stomach (yang), the lungs (yin) with the large intestine (yang), the heart (yin) with the small intestine (yang), and the pericardium, the sac around the heart, (yin) with the triple heater (yang). The two other meridians described as major channels not connected with particular organs run along the center of the torso and together control the yin and yang of the whole body. They are called the Governor Vessel and the Conception Vessel.

There are five regular yin meridian organ pairs (Kidney, Liver, Spleen, Lung, and Heart) connected with five basic emotions that directly affect how we experience our world. Each intense emotion we feel directly affects our meridians and organs, impacting how they function. (In the future, when I refer to kidney or liver, for example, I mean the meridian-organ functions together.) When out of balance, the kidneys are linked with fear and terror, the liver with anger and envy, the spleen with obsession and worry, the lungs with sadness and grief, and the heart with hatred or depression. Unbalanced and excessive emotions lead to illness and disease just as undernourished organs and depleted chi promote disturbing emotions. A regular Yin/Yang yoga practice can stimulate the flow of chi in these electromagnetic routes (meridians), enhancing each organ's function, relieving energetic and emotional blockages in the meridians, and generating a fresh aliveness in how we think and feel. With its quiet atmosphere unstained by striving, the Yin practice in particular allows us the space to fully metabolize emotions we often ingest but cannot completely digest. In the following chapters, I will describe the importance of each meridian-organ pair for overall health and outline four Yin sequences to revitalize and restore vibrancy to each. As there are only a dozen or so Yin poses that nourish the deeper meridians well, you will see a repetition of these poses placed in varying sequences to create specific amplifications. Each pose affects many meridians, but I have listed a specific meridian pair in each chapter that will be benefited most by the specific sequence offered.

6

The Kidneys and Urinary Bladder

THE KIDNEY-BLADDER pairs of meridians and organs in Chinese medicine are the foundation of Yin-and-Yang balance for all the other organs. Like primordial parents, they are fundamental for birth, metamorphosis, and reproduction. The Kidney meridian flows up the interior and center of the body, while the Urinary Bladder meridian flows down the entire back of the body, and the kidney organ opens into the bladder. They are a storehouse of vital energy and need to remain balanced for all the other organs to function well. It is for this reason that I have begun the discussion of organ health and Yin yoga with them and recommend that you begin your practice with the kidney poses and come back to these sequences often throughout your life. In Chinese medicine, the kidneys are considered the officials of the energetic work. Although the yin/yang teams of organs in the following chapters on specific organ-meridian pairs have different anatomical functions, most of their energetic and mental qualities are so similar that I have only described their unique physical characteristics separately, while the remaining characteristics listed in each chapter refer to both kidney/bladder energetic qualities or spleen/stomach mental qualities, and so on.

Physical Qualities
Kidneys

The kidneys are located at about waist height, behind the lower ribs. They filter fifteen gallons of blood an hour, purifying it and breaking it down into nutritional elements for the body. They are in charge of balancing bodily fluids and regulating blood pressure and glucose metabolism. When this function is interrupted, we see high blood pressure, hypertension, and toxicity in the body, as well as an achy lower abdomen, swelling and bloating, and difficulty in urinating. Lower body circulation will also be poor.

Bladder

The kidneys open up into the bladder, which is the complementary yang organ. It is the storage site for urine through which we eliminate fluid waste. The bladder is quite flexible and can contain a little or a lot, a function that relates not only to a physical capacity but mental flexibility as well. The Urinary Bladder (UB) meridian is the longest in the body and has sixty-seven acupuncture points along it, making it a superhighway in the meridian system. Most notably, it is the only meridian of the fourteen main channels, besides the Governor Vessel, that flows through the brain.

Energetic Qualities
Kidney-Bladder Organ-Meridian Pair

> The Kidneys are the mansion of Fire and Water, the residence of *yin* and *yang* . . . the channel of life and death. They link the past and the future. —Francesca Diebschlag

According to Chinese medicine, the kidneys house our essence energy, or jing. It is considered the substance that pervades all organic life and is the essence of growth and decline. It is connected to our ancestry, our inherited constitution, and our capacity for differentiation into yin and yang. It is the underlying material of each organ's substance, bestowing the capacity for life activity.

Jing rules the production of bone marrow as well as bone development and repair. Bone marrow is a soft, fatty material that is lighter than actual bone and fills the hollow bones in the skull, vertebrae, and ribs, as well as those in children's extremities. It is in the bone marrow that we produce blood cells. The red blood cells are generated within our round bones and carry oxygen, while the white blood cells produced in our flat bones assist with immune response. If kidney jing is deficient in children, their bones may become soft, whereas in adults, we see problems with the skeleton or poor immune functions.

While the kidneys are the storage containers for our essence energy, their energetic health rules the general health of the lower back, the reproductive organs, the urinary system, the lower intestinal tract, and all the fluid systems of the body, including the joint lubrication. If we suffer from a fragile back, have had back injuries or weakness, or feel pain coming from this area even when the muscles are not engaged, we can be sure we have kidney issues. We may repeatedly injure our lower back and hope that the simple remedy is to strengthen our abdominals and back muscles, but the deeper cure is to strengthen our kidney chi.

The kidneys also act as step-up transformers when our energy is low, working overtime when we are stressed, overcommitted, or continuing to push on even though we are exhausted. Learning to cultivate appropriate rhythms and live a life in balance is essential for the health of our kidneys and all our other organs as well.

In the five-element theory, the kidneys are closest to the element of water and are connected to all the systems of flow within us. Since the body is composed of approximately 60 to 70 percent water, fluid bathes the entire cellular system, and the health of the kidneys directly impacts the moisture content of all of our fluid systems. This includes the blood and circulatory system, lymphatic system, endocrine system, urinary system, perspiration, saliva, tears, sexual secretions, and lactation.

If we have a lot of upper body heat as a result of our constitution or lifestyle, the heat of the fire energy will weaken the kidneys, breaking down our energy balance, and causing health problems. The more heat in the stomach, the more the kidneys are weakened. This means someone with a lot of inner fire who also eats spicy foods and does a hot (Yang) yoga practice with lots of poses for the upper body will compromise the kidneys' ability to balance the body with cool moisture. The circulation in the lower body will also be poor if there is excess heat in the stomach, causing the energy of the kidneys to be overpowered.

Passive, Yin-style straddle splits (dragonfly pose) that pull on the inner thighs and long-held backbends that lengthen the anterior (front of the) spine and compress the posterior side, stimulating the chi through the longitudinal ligaments, are a wonderful way to nourish kidney chi. This helps diminish excess heat in the body, while also enhancing the cooling capacity of the kidneys. The kidney chi is connected to our sense of hearing and corresponds to the ears.

Emotional Qualities

Staying still in various poses will undoubtedly bring up lots of emotions. As we surrender into the sensations, we have the opportunity to acknowledge all that arises within us, allowing ourselves time to fully inhabit our emotions, without the compulsion to act out because of them.

We may experience disappointment in a tight hip or fear as we settle into a long-held backbend. The longer we practice, the more we notice how varied our feelings are, how we can feel agitation one minute and elation the next, exuberance followed by despair. Inside the cocoon of long-held poses, we can turn toward these various nuances, and track our passing states of being. This breeds an emotional flexibility and resiliency.

Often, our uninvestigated habit may be to feel defeated or oppressed by disturbing emotions, immediately identifying with them. With practice, we can instead learn to soften into the resistance or anguish and truly examine its momentum. Whatever the content, we train ourselves to open to the experience. This capacity to remain attentive and nonjudgmental toward what we are experiencing naturally transforms the experience from one of struggling with difficulty to one of opening up to challenges. What results is not an increase in suffering, as we may initially fear, but more openness.

There is a common misconception that we should be able to control or eradicate pain. Although yoga poses do often bring some relief to blocked areas of the body, we will still have to endure discomforting pains as long as we are in this body. Instead of expecting to miraculously become pain free from a yoga practice, we can utilize the poses to help us fully inhabit our bodies with dignity and care, whether we are experiencing pleasure or pain.

If we want to learn how to come home to our bodies, we have to take up residence in every corner of ourselves, no matter how sick, injured, decrepit, or immobile we are. Each Yin pose is another opportunity to crawl into ourselves and stay a while. While remaining still, we allow ourselves to breathe into our feeling tones without the burden of expecting to feel a particular way or create a particular result.

Some days I notice feelings of discontent and restlessness. Time and time again, I am amazed that even a few moments of letting myself open up, without judgment, to however I am feeling has a

therapeutic and refreshing effect on my body and mind. I have learned these moods are like passing clouds that needn't be pushed away or clung to.

I particularly remember the afternoon of 9/11. My sister lived very close to the twin towers, and I was full of disbelief, anger, anxiety, and anguish. Having listened to the news commentators all morning, I was feeling both overwhelmed and exhausted. By afternoon, I felt a bit numb and depleted. I needed to retreat from all the information filling the airwaves. I plopped down in the sun in my living room and started holding various Yin poses. Even as I swirled in incredulity, raged and wept, I felt a healing capacity emerging the longer I practiced. Abiding in a soft practice while experiencing all the shifting emotions felt like the most loving act I could perform at that moment. I emerged after an hour sobered, strengthened, and surprisingly prepared to go out that evening and teach the beginning of a course on yin and mindfulness. I do not think I would have had the physical or emotional strength to provide a supportive atmosphere to allow others to grieve and digest their emotions that day if I had not had a practice that affects the confluence of the body, emotions, and states of mind.

In Chinese medicine, the emotions are simply an expression of chi and are not considered good or bad. It is less important which emotions are present and more about whether they are able to flow without impediment, whether they are blocked or repressed. Every prolonged disturbing emotion affects the heath of our organs and meridians, and every imbalance in our organ-meridian system is tied to a propensity for certain emotions. When the kidneys are out of balance, the main emotional flavor is fear. We may hold on to things and people with a marked fear of letting go or an overall lack of trust, both in ourselves and in others. Kidney chi imbalance is associated with all kinds of fears, such as a fear of heights, water, people, new places, sexuality, being taken advantage of, and death. As these are fears common to us all, it is helpful to know that when we are consumed by a constricting presence of fear, we tax our kidney energy, and if our kidney chi is deficient, we will feel fearful more easily. It works both ways.

Conversely, when our kidney chi is balanced, we will experience an emotional capacity to access our innate gentleness, openness, and ultimately, our primordial wisdom. But just to be clear, the organs do not cause emotions, as all emotions stem from the heart and are drawn to different organs, which can damage them.

If we are trying to determine which organ an emotion comes from, the answer will always be the same: all emotions originate in the heart. Chapter eight of the *Su Wen* states, "The heart holds the office of monarch, whence the spirit light (*shen ming*) originates." If we think of this "spirit light" as consciousness, we can say that all of our emotions originate from within our consciousness. So long as the heart and its consciousness are functioning normally, the emotions will remain peaceful, like a well-governed country.

—*Yong Ping Jiang, DOM, PhD*

When we experience an energetic ease of being, the Yin sessions can help maintain and build on these intrinsic capacities. When we do not feel this way, settling into these long-held poses can allow us to identify our reactive emotions, such as fear, and investigate them in a nourishing way. We learn that we can relax our resistance to strong sensations and emotions, turning toward—rather than away from—what is arising within us. This classic mindful approach neutralizes the destructive side of an emotion by observing an emotion's movement without compulsively acting it out. This is simply called participatory observation.

For example, while holding a backbend, we may experience alarm as the minutes progress and we feel the sensations of compression in our lumbar spine. As we rest the mind on the sensations in our back and allow the feeling of trepidation to move through us, we literally give our inner life more space to be just as it is, without mental constriction. As a result, a curious thing occurs. The original feeling of something like fear is now also permeated with attention, producing a feeling of alert allowance.

From this vantage point, we can authentically investigate the anatomy of any emotion. As we develop a keen sense of witnessing our patterns of behavior, we can examine the whole mechanism that occurs within us. Fear is not a static thing we can label. Under scrutiny, we may notice fear is supported by a collage of sensations rising and falling, as well as streams of inner dialogue left uninvestigated, often hardening into assumed truths. The generous time we spend in each pose allows us to penetrate these emotional blocks with care. Since we have no agenda to uphold during these five-minute intervals, our inward-drawn attention allows them to simply move through us.

When we question the stories we are telling ourselves and stay with the process of naked observation, intuitions and insights that have been shrouded by our fears are given the opportunity to filter through. While continuing to relax into the pose, we create what Buddhist psychiatrist Mark Epstein calls "a holding environment" inside ourselves. Like an understanding parent relating to a difficult teen by neither abandoning them nor antagonizing them, we create space for our fear to exist, free of the harness of resistance. The habit and strong compulsion to defend, deny, or act out from these feelings is what causes the torment, not the feelings themselves.

As we quietly observe our feelings rise and fall inside us, we begin to relate to them like the breath, giving them space to move. As a result, we feel them like waves on the ocean, rising up, peaking, and eventually subsiding. We may start our session with a cacophony of difficult emotions pouring through us, but as our moments unfold and we neither repress nor react from states such as fear, we learn to live in the direct experience of meditative awareness of the body, heart, and mind. Awareness is our greatest security and foundation for emotional maturity.

Mental Qualities

The kidneys are associated with short-term memory, willpower, and healthy ambition. If our kidney energy is deficient, we have trouble completing tasks, have less energetic and sexual drive, and feel less enthusiasm to follow through on our plans. We may experience ourselves with a diminished sense of personal power and feel disconnected inside. As our energy is already depleted, we do not feel that we can pull ourselves out of this malaise. We haven't the energy to do so, and our thoughts may spiral in circles of confusion. As studies at the National Institutes of Health have determined, when we have a negative thought and don't challenge it, our minds believe it and our brains react to it. This causes a whole psychosomatic spiral that can lead to despair, anguish, and ill health.

Yin practice can be very helpful in these times because it does not require energetic effort to get our body into these shapes. As we let go into the poses, we have an opportunity to view the content of our minds from a fresh perspective. We can then begin to acknowledge the voices that come from our reactive patterns and believe in them less. We learn to watch our thoughts come and go, relaxing our assumptions that what we tell ourselves is the incontestable truth. To develop this capacity of inner listening, we simply need to come to the floor and be willing to turn our attention toward our physical and psychological experience with care.

Just as stated for the kidneys, an imbalance in the UB channel is connected with an inability to cope with life and fear of change, two serious impediments to well-being. The Kidney and UB meridian organs' influence on our body-mind is connected with the limbic system housed near the center of the brain.

The limbic system performs a number of crucial functions, including controlling sleep cycles, appetite, and libido; promoting bonding; modulating motivation; and setting the emotional tone of the mind, providing a filter through which external experiences are integrated into emotional states. It marks specific events as internally important and accumulates our intense emotional memories. Problems with the limbic system are indicated by excessive moodiness, irritability (also connected with heart meridian-organ functions), negative thinking, and clinical depression, as well as an inability to make plans, solve problems, or organize (also connected with liver chi function).

The limbic system's power to control mood and attitude adds both the positive and the negative emotional flavor that is considered critical for survival. The total experience of our emotional memories is responsible for our emotional tone of mind, so the more steady positive experiences we have, the more optimistic we are able to feel. Emotional traumas such as abuse, accidents, and catastrophies are also stored in the deep limbic system, and these experiences tend to color our capacity for future ease of being.

Neuroscientists suggest that the limbic system needs to be kept cool and underactive in order for us to feel emotionally stable. When it is inflamed and overactive, negative emotional shading results. With a heated-up limbic system, we are more likely to interpret a neutral or even a positive event in a negative way. Studies have shown that the deep limbic system becomes more active and inflamed during women's hormonal cycles, including puberty, menstruation, pregnancy, childbirth, lactation, and menopause. This time of overactivity is associated with depression and anxiety.

Having a meditation and Yin yoga practice that allows us to relax muscular tension and observe our inner atmosphere by diving into a contemplative attitude can begin to calm the central nervous system and cool the limbic system during these times. If we also take poses that stimulate the nourishment of the Kidney and UB meridians (that flow through the brain), we accelerate the chemical and attitudinal balance we need. Our practice can be a place where we create positive experiences to store in the limbic system's emotional memory by inviting challenging circumstances (holding a yin pose) while we relax our struggle with whatever emotional difficulty we are facing. This quality of allowance increases our capacity to stay compassionately attuned to our sensations and feelings without insisting any improvement occur, diminishing our tension within. In Yin practice, we are carving out neural pathways of loving-kindness toward ourselves as we learn to feel deeply into our bodies just as they are.

What follows in chapter 7 is an effective combination of useful poses to boost kidney chi and organ health. As you may be quite drained at times when you come to do this practice, please remain extra-sensitive and respect your natural limitations. You need not impose an ambitious agenda on yourself with regard to how much sensation you should be able to tolerate or how long you think you ought to be able to stay in each pose. The Yin practice is a time for revitalizing your depleted chi. There is no need to force, strain, rush, fix, or in any way struggle with yourself right now. It is the attitude of relaxed attention that begins the process of renourishing your being on many levels.

Yin Yoga and Pregnancy

Once upon a time it was thought that pregnant women were fragile. They were discouraged by doctors and concerned fathers from doing any exercise or exerting themselves in any way. It is now understood that pregnant women are capable of doing nearly everything that every other woman is capable of, and in some cases more. Today, pregnant women are emphatically encouraged to do yoga as it has shown to ease the physical and emotional rigors of labor and increase the overall sense of well-being through the many transitions of motherhood.

Yin yoga can be geared toward pregnancy quite easily as long as the expectant mother is guided to stretch conservatively to take into account that she has an increased amount of the hormones elastin and relaxin (joint laxity), which causes more elasticity in the joints. This can be a danger because she might not feel discomfort even when overstretching and she could strain her joints as a result. We all need to listen to the feedback from our body, and that feedback might feel different during pregnancy. As with any physical practice, it is important that a pregnant woman consult her healthcare practitioner before beginning an exercise program, including Yin yoga.

Among the many benefits to doing a Yin practice while pregnant is that the poses stimulate the tissues to help create more fluid mobility throughout the system, increasing the comfort in the body as it grows and changes. Stimulating the meridians in this way also contributes to a healthier organ system, another plus, because the organs are working harder during pregnancy and lactation. Because the practice serves as a needleless acupuncture session, it can help balance a woman's overall energy and emotions, which are naturally destabilized by the hormone infusion during this time. Last, but perhaps the most important reason to practice this style while pregnant is the meditative atmosphere it creates. I feel that learning or continuing to deepen into mindfulness meditation during pregnancy is of utmost importance. In pregnancy as in motherhood, we are called on to ride the erratic emotions triggered by hormones. We need to be able to flow with difficult circumstances without enduring prolonged inward rigidity and tension, which have a direct and immediate impact on the fetus and child. We can't prevent this reactivity from arising, but we can temper it by relating to difficult emotions consciously in our daily practice. With a mindfulness meditation practice, we learn to suspend the compulsion to lash out when we are triggered, upset, or just plain tired.

I am immensely grateful to my committed yoga and meditation practices, as they have been utterly invaluable to me throughout my pregnancy and motherhood.

7

Yin Yoga Sequences for the Kidneys and Urinary Bladder

The Kidney and Urinary Bladder Meridians

THE KIDNEY MERIDIAN begins at the little toe in each foot, running through the sole, through the arch, and up the inside of the knees and legs, entering the torso near the tailbone. It moves up along the longitudinal ligaments of the lower spine, connecting internally with the bladder and kidneys. It also moves externally over the abdomen and chest, while internally flowing through the liver, diaphragm, and lungs. It goes through the throat and ends at the root of the tongue. These meridians often have several branches and run through both legs or arms even when drawn through only one. The solid lines are meridians that run closer to the surface, and the broken lines are in the center.

The Urinary Bladder meridian starts at the inside of the eyes, goes up the forehead and across the crown, and enters the brain. It then runs down the back body parallel to the spine. A branch goes into the body at the lumbar spine and connects with the kidneys and urinary bladder. Outer branches run all the way down the backs of the legs and end at the little toes.

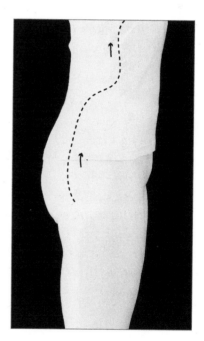

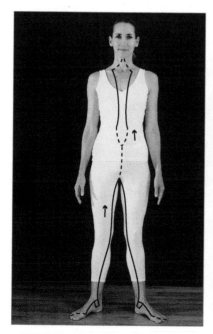

The Kidney Meridian

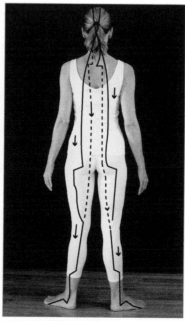

The Urinary Bladder Meridian

The Kidney Meridian, side view

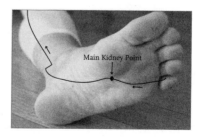

The Kidney Meridian, K1 point

Kidney/Urinary Bladder Short Session

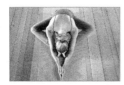 Butterfly Pose, or Lying Butterfly Pose

 Saddle Pose, or Sphinx Pose

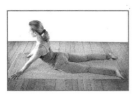 Seal Pose, or Sphinx Pose

 Child's Pose

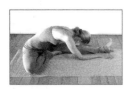 Half-Dragonfly Pose, or Legs-Up-the-Wall Pose

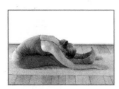 Full Forward Bend

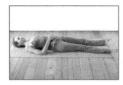 Corpse Pose (Savasana)

Butterfly Pose

This pose stimulates the Kidney meridian as it flows along the inner legs and through the torso (Fig. 7.1).

Begin by sitting on the floor with equal weight in both sitting bones (slightly elevated on a cushion or rolled up blanket) and your spine upright with your legs extended. Bending your knees, bring the soles of the feet together with your hands on your ankles. Move your feet forward so that your legs form a diamond shape. As your knees drop out to the side like butterfly wings, let your weight shift to the front edge of your sitting bones. (If you have any disc displacements, suffer from sciatica, or have strained your sacroiliac region in the past, you may want to stay upright or rest back in Lying Butterfly Pose, described next).

If you have a weak or injured knee or hip, place a cushion under the corresponding thigh(s) for support. With your hands on your ankles, start to bend forward from the hips until you feel an appropriate amount of stretch in the tissues of your outer hip, inner groin, and lower back. As you bend forward, let your back relax into the fold, allowing your head to rest either into the arches of your feet, on top of your stacked fists, or cupped in your hands while your elbows rest on your feet. You may also rest on top of a bolster or pillow (Fig. 7.2).

Remember the three principles of a Yin practice. First, come into the pose to your appropriate

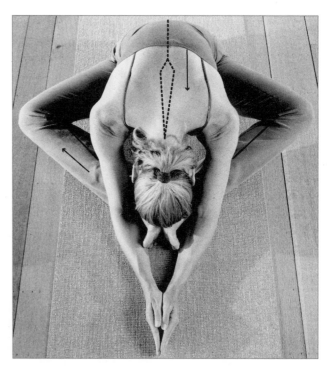

7.1. Butterfly Pose—Kidney meridian shown

edge, allowing stimulating sensations to be present without feeling overwhelmed or alarmed. Second, become still, muscularly unengaged but stretched, and mentally willing to surrender to the experience. Third, hold the pose for a while. I recommend 3 to 5 minutes to start, but if one minute is enough for you, start with that; in a month or so, work up to 2 minutes.

To come out, inhale as you bring your spine slowly back to an upright position. Slowly stretch your legs out in front of you and rest back on your hands. Each time you end a pose that you've held for several minutes, pause a few moments in a neutral position such as this to allow your body to effortlessly nourish the area you have just emphasized.

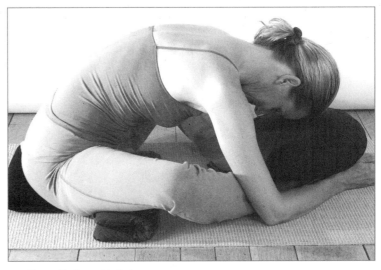

7.2. Butterfly Pose, Variation 1

Lying Butterfly Pose

Follow the instructions for Butterfly Pose, bringing your feet together and dropping your knees out to the sides. Instead of folding forward, rest back on your elbows or a bolster, or lie back on pillows or on the floor with your hands on your abdomen (Fig. 7.3). You can also place pillows under the thighs for added support if you have a tight groin or sensitive knees.

Saddle Pose

This pose stimulates the Kidney meridian-organ as it flows through the sacrolumbar area and the longitudinal ligaments along the lumbar spine, as well as the kidneys themselves (Fig. 7.4).

Begin by sitting on your feet with your knees in full flexion and slightly apart; lean back on your hands. If this is too much for your knees, you can substitute Saddle for Sphinx Pose instead (see description on page 41). Allow your lower back to form an exaggerated arch as you lean back, tilting your sacrum toward your lumbar spine. If it does not strain your quadriceps, come down onto your elbows or upper back. You can also rest back on a bolster, but I suggest placing it under your shoulders and leaving your lower back unsupported (Fig. 7.5) to ask more of these tissues by stressing them appropriately. If you have any disc displacement or injury, it is advisable to place the

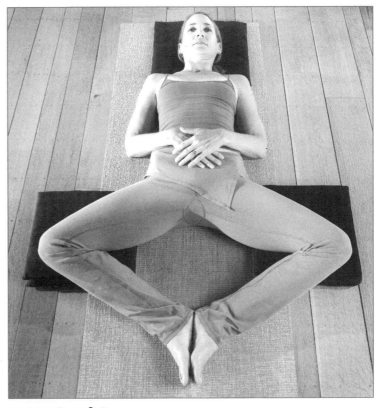

7.3. Lying Butterfly Pose

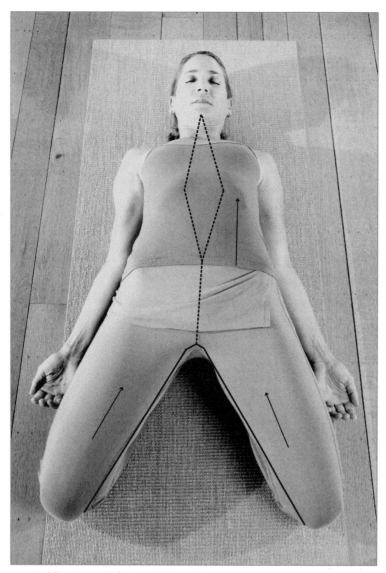

7.4. Saddle Pose—Kidney meridian shown

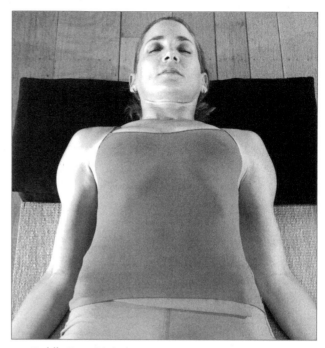

7.5. Saddle Pose, Variation 1

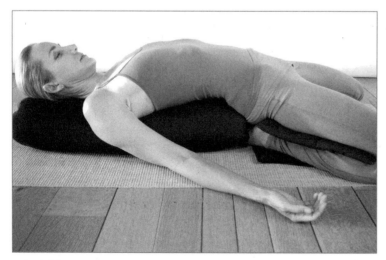

7.6. Saddle Pose, Variation 2

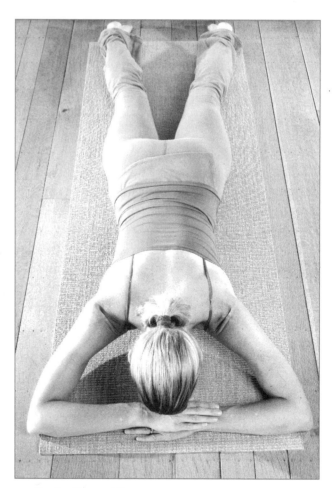

7.7. Resting Forward Pose

bolster lengthwise, beginning at your sacrum, to support your whole spine (Fig. 7.6). You can also lessen the flexion in the knees by placing a rolled blanket in the back crease of the knees. For tight ankles, place a cushion between your ankles and the floor.

If you find the pose too difficult at this point but can flex your knees quite a bit, you can alter the sequence and do Dragon Pose (see description on page 76) on each leg first; add Half-Saddle Pose next (see page 79), then attempt full Saddle Pose.

Allow your knees to rest comfortably apart. There is no need to try and keep them together, as this will stress them and/or your sacrum if you are more externally rotated. If your head is not resting on the floor or a cushion and your cervical spine is healthy, you can drop your head back for some or all of the time. If your neck feels fragile or is weak, then keep your chin tilted toward your chest and your head in line with your spine.

Stay in the pose for 3 to 5 minutes. To come out, place your hands next to your sides where your elbows have been. On an inhalation, engage your abdominal muscles and come up in the same way you went back. (This is safer than sliding your legs out from under you.) Since you have been resting your back muscles passively for several minutes, it is important to engage your abdominals to assist in your ascent so your back does not try and do this on its own. Lie on your belly with your legs outstretched for a moment (Fig. 7.7) before proceeding to the next pose.

Sphinx Pose

This pose stimulates the Kidney meridian-organ as it flows through the sacrolumbar area and the longitudinal ligaments along the lumbar spine (Fig. 7.8).

Lie on your belly. Push up to rest on your elbows, which should be shoulder-width apart and positioned an inch or so forward of the shoulder line. (If they are too far back, your shoulders will start to feel quite heavy.) Bring your palms together in front of you or cross your arms and let your hands rest on your elbows. Allow yourself to rest upright, without slumping into your shoulders

or attempting to lift up from them. Your back will arch in a gentle sway that creates length along the anterior of your spine and gentle compression on the posterior side. You can allow your buttocks and legs to relax as long as you feel no sharp or shooting pains. If you do, move your elbows farther forward so your ribs also carry some of your weight, and engage your inner thighs (Fig. 7.9). This will allow your back to maintain a very gentle arch, without straining your limited range of motion.

Passive backbends stimulate kidney chi, revitalizing your energy supply, so allow your belly and organs to drape toward the floor and relax your buttocks and legs. However, if your back

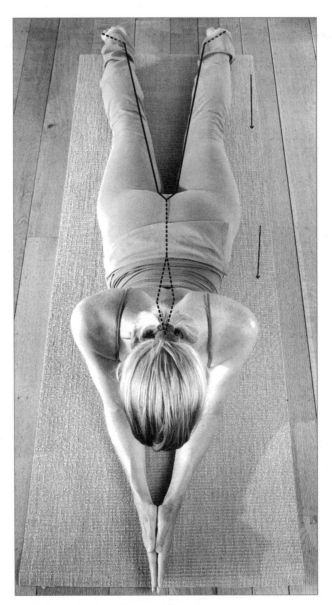

7.8. Sphinx Pose—Kidney meridian shown

currently has sensitivities, you can engage the muscles in your outer buttocks and inner legs all or part of the time to relieve the strong sensations occurring in the ligaments along your spine. If you would like to intensify this backbend a bit, place a cushion under your elbows (Fig. 7.10).

Stay in the pose for 3 to 5 minutes. To come out, on an exhalation, slowly move your elbows out to the sides and lower your upper body to the floor. Rest in this lying position for a minute or so.

When it feels appropriate to move again, place your hands under your chest, and on an inhalation, slowly push your upper body away from the floor. As you exhale, settle your hips back toward your feet in Child's Pose (Fig. 7.11).

Child's Pose

Kneel with your back straight and your feet pointing in toward each other, arms at your sides. Sit back by moving your hips toward your feet, your knees slightly apart, and your head relaxing toward the floor. Your hands can either rest down by your sides or stack them like a pillow under your forehead. Stay for 1–2 minutes.

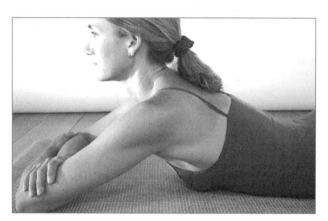

7.9. Sphinx Pose, Variation 1

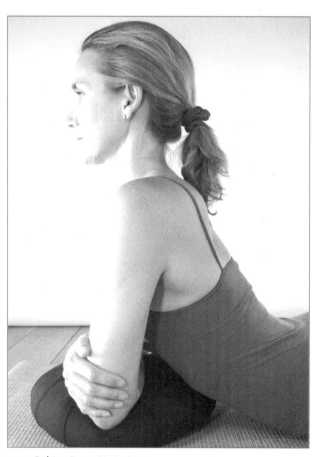

7.10. Sphinx Pose, Variation 2

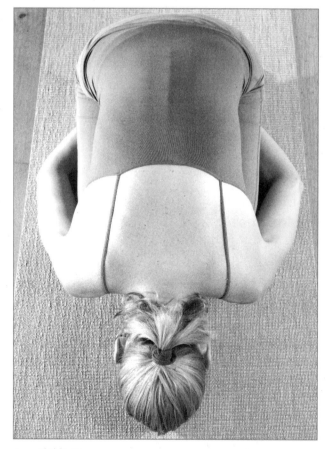

7.11. Child's Pose

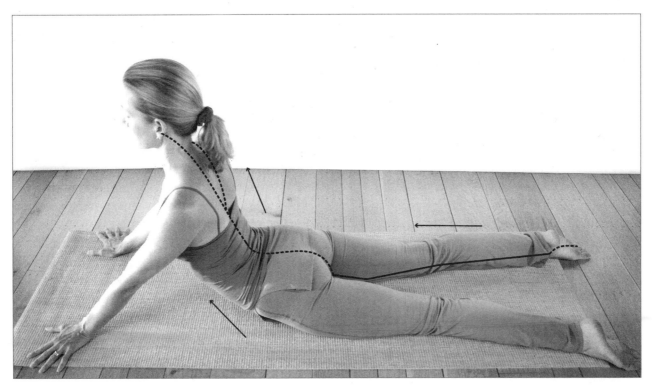

7.12. Seal Pose—Kidney meridian shown

Seal Pose

This pose is similar to Sphinx Pose but causes more compression on the lower back and may not be suitable for everyone. If this is too difficult, do Sphinx Pose instead. It stimulates the Kidney meridian as it flows through the sacrolumbar area and the longitudinal ligaments along the lumbar spine (Fig. 7.12).

To begin, lie on your belly with your hands out in front of you. As you inhale, using your back muscles, slide your hands closer in toward your body until they are about 4 inches in front of your shoulders with your arms straight. (Note: You use your arms like posts in this pose, but if you have hypermobile elbows, be sure to allow some flexion or a slight bend to avoid locking the elbows.) You can turn your hands outward slightly, like a seal's flippers. Be sure to maintain an even distribution of weight across both hands to avoid overstressing portions of your wrists.

Your spine will be in a dramatic backbend, with the stress of the pose targeting your sacrolumbar region. Keep your head upright and in line with your spine for optimal neck comfort. (Note: Some people enjoy dropping their head back at times during the pose, stimulating the cervical vertebrae, but this can create neck strain if it is held too long.)

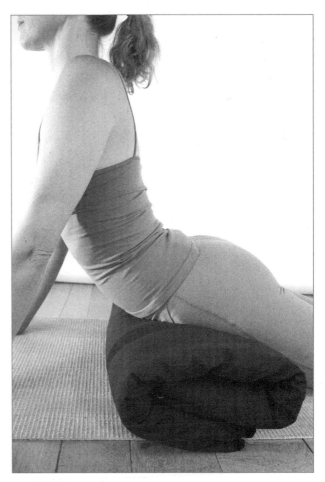

7.13. Seal Pose, Variation 1

As was mentioned for Sphinx Pose, you can either allow the muscles in your buttocks and legs to relax, if this is comfortable, or alternate contracting and releasing them to relieve some of the intense sensations. It may take a few months of consistent practice for you to develop healthier lower back tissues and increase your ability to remain muscularly soft in this pose. Be patient and do not endure so much sensation that you cannot breathe easily or that you feel stressed while in the pose.

Remember, the Yin poses can be very beneficial during pregnancy as long as we do not go to our deepest edge in each pose, as we have more elasticity in the joints when pregnant. If you are pregnant or would like to maintain this dramatic backbend while easing the feelings of compression in your lower back, place a folded blanket under your pubic bones (Fig. 7.13).

Stay in this pose for 3 to 5 minutes if you can do so without distress. Otherwise, begin with 1 to 2 minutes in Seal Pose and then continue in Sphinx Pose for a few more minutes.

To come out, on an exhalation, bend your elbows to lower yourself slowly. Remain still, lying on your belly and continuing to breathe into your whole spine as you rest. Notice the change in sensations now that you have come out of this intense pose. You may detect cooling sensations, inner feelings of refreshment, or a restful calm. Allow yourself to absorb these fully before slowly moving to Child's Pose.

Half-Dragonfly Pose

This pose stimulates the Bladder meridian-organ as it flows down the back of your body and the backs of your legs (Fig. 7.14).

Sit straight and bring your right foot in near your pelvis. Bring your right hip and knee further over to the right (as much as you can), yet turn the torso to face the left leg. Take a breath in and, as you exhale, begin to tilt your hips forward. (You can also elevate your sitting bones on a cushion as you did in Butterfly Pose if you have tight hamstrings or lower back muscles.)

Note: Many people wonder if it is all right to round the back in this pose. The spinal ligaments will actually be more affected if you curve the spine, as this creates a stronger pull on the tissues. There are a couple of exceptions to this. One is that you do not want to fold your upper body forward to the point of collapsing your chest, because this may tense and shrink the space around your diaphragm and hinder your breathing. Try to allow your spine to round as you come forward while maintaining

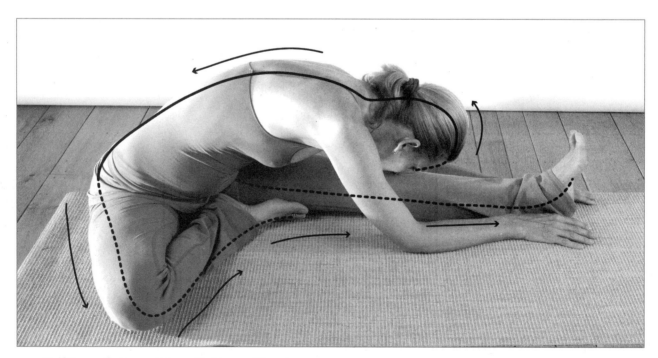

7.14. Half-Dragonfly Pose—Urinary Bladder meridian shown

a sense of frontal space and ease around your diaphragm. The other case in which folding forward is counterproductive is if you already have an exaggerated curve in your thoracic spine, a condition called kyphosis. If you do, it is helpful to avoid long-held forward bends altogether and instead you can do Legs-Up-the-Wall Pose (described next).

Place your hands on the floor and then slide down till they are on either side of your foot, as in the photo. Once you feel your natural limitation preventing you from bending any more, allow yourself to remain steady in a nonaggressive way, neither pulling yourself farther down nor strongly engaging your leg muscles. If you have any knee issues, you can hold this pose with your quadriceps firm and simply allow your back muscles to pull you forward naturally. You may need to put a cushion under your right (bent) knee if it is not resting on the floor or if it feels sensitive in any way (Fig. 7.15).

If you have sciatica or a pulled hamstring, you should place a cushion under your left (extended) knee to prevent full extension in the leg.

Alternatively, for tight or overstressed hamstrings you can bend your left knee, placing a cushion underneath it for support, and put the sole of your foot on the floor before folding forward (Fig. 7.16).

You can support your head if you like by resting your elbows on the floor on either side of your knee and holding your chin in your palms (see Fig. 7.15). Some people like to rest their forehead on their stacked fists or place a cushion under their forehead (Fig. 7.17). Placing padding under the extended knee is helpful for tight or overstressed hamstrings.

If your cervical spine is healthy, it is fine to simply hang your head forward without support. If your neck has been through some trauma or has a diminished natural curve (or a reversed curve), then using one of the suggested supports is safer.

Stay in the pose for 3 to 5 minutes. To come out, raise up on an inhalation, slowly stacking your vertebrae one by one until you are upright. Stretch both legs out in front of you and lean back on your hands for a moment, sensitizing yourself to the sensation of chi migrating down into your left leg.

This pose stimulates the Urinary Bladder channels that run down both sides of your back, along either side of your spine, and down into the backs of your legs. Remember that whatever you do to your

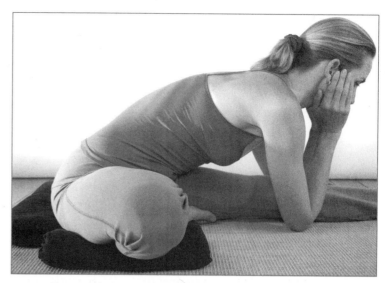

7.15. Half-Dragonfly Pose, Variation 1

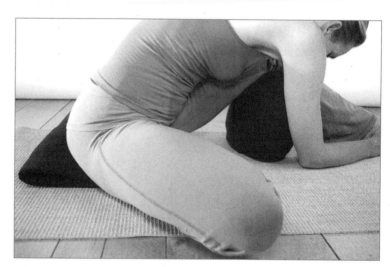

7.16. Half-Dragonfly Pose, Variation 2

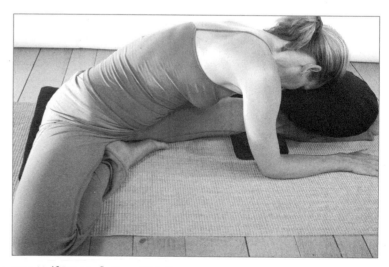

7.17. Half-Dragonfly Pose, Variation 3

bladder meridian immediately affects your Kidney channels and vice versa, so this forward bend is not only an intelligent counterpose to the passive back-bends that came earlier, but a complementary way to further enhance your kidney chi. After pausing a moment or two, repeat the pose with your left foot pulled in and your right leg extended.

Legs-Up-the-Wall Pose

Sit straight with your right hip touching a wall and your legs straight out in front of you. As you lie back, swivel around and slide your legs up the wall; this should allow you to position yourself right up with your buttocks against the wall when you are lying flat (Fig. 7.18). Keep your sacrum weighted toward the floor, and rest your head back so that your chin is at about the same height as your forehead. If it feels higher, place a folded blanket under your head only. If your legs feel like they will bend easily

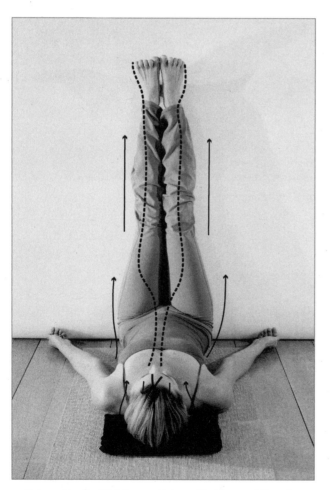

7.18. Legs-Up-the-Wall Pose—Urinary Bladder meridian shown

and cause your feet to slide down the wall, wrap a strap around your thighs just above your knees.

Stay in this pose for 3 to 5 minutes. This position causes the typical downward pull of chi (which often pools and stagnates in your legs) to be reversed, refreshing the circulation throughout your lower body meridians. To come out, bend the knees and either push with your feet away from the wall or twist to the side and use your hands to sit up.

Full Forward Bend

This pose stimulates the Bladder meridian as it flows down the back of your body and backs of your legs (Fig. 7.19).

As in all forward bends, you can place a cushion under the sitting bones if you have tight hamstrings or lower back muscles. With your sitting bones on a slightly raised cushion, begin to bend forward from the hips, allowing your spine to curve into a forward bend. (Please review the note about appropriate spinal curve in forward bends under Half-Dragonfly Pose. The suggestions about knee and head support apply in this pose as well.) If you have sciatica and find that full forward bends cause your hips to tilt away from your legs, i.e., in retroversion—often because of tight hamstrings and/or lower back muscles—or you experience pain in your spine after performing these poses, bend both knees and put your feet flat on the floor next to each other; you may wish to put a rolled blanket or bolster under your knees for support (Fig. 7.20).

When you bend your knees, it is much easier to bend forward from the hips, which will give a nice stretch to your lower back without leg and/or hip issues restricting your movement as much. If you have pulled a hamstring in the past, it is best to keep your knees slightly flexed by placing a pad under them in this pose (Fig. 7.21).

If you need support for your neck, rest your forehead on a cushion placed on your legs (Fig. 7.22).

You can eliminate this pose if your front hip bones do not tilt forward in Full Forward Bends and the above suggestions do not cause this to occur. In that case, you can do Legs-Up-the-Wall Pose instead.

Stay in this pose for 3 to 5 minutes. To come out, on an inhalation, raise your spine slowly, stacking your vertebrae one by one until you're

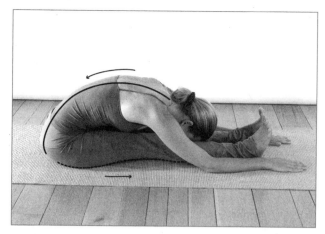

7.19. Full Forward Bend—Urinary Bladder meridian shown

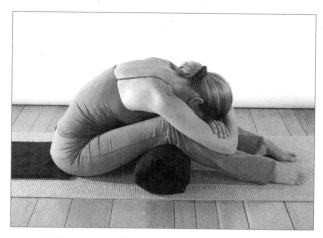

7.20. Full Forward Bend, Variation 1

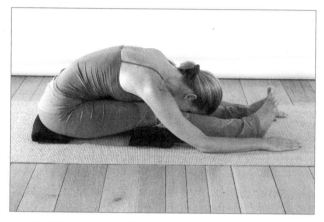

7.21. Full Forward Bend, Variation 2

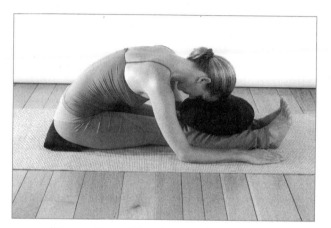

7.22. Full Forward Bend, Variation 3

upright. Allow yourself to rest back on your hands again for a moment, aware of the feeling of chi coursing through your hips and into your legs like a newly installed irrigation system.

As mentioned for Half-Dragonfly Pose, straight-leg forward bends stimulate the Urinary Bladder channels that intersect with the kidneys, allowing for the dual effect of both calming (remember that the Urinary Bladder meridian is the only one besides the Governor Vessel meridian that runs through the brain) and reenergizing the system. Lie back in this state of restful refreshment.

Corpse Pose (Savasana)

As you lie on your back, keep your shoulder blades down away from your ears and rest your hands on your abdomen (Fig. 7.23). Alternately, you can allow your arms to rest away from your body with the palms facing up (Fig. 7.24).

Move your head gently from side to side to find a balance of weight on the back of your head. Move your legs apart wider than your hips, and allow your buttocks, legs, and feet to relax completely. Feel as if you have been carrying around a heavy load that you've just let drop to the floor. Don't move your body or your mind now. Relax your attention with the sensations of pulsation undulating throughout your being. This vibration is the formless chi body, and fine-tuning your sensitivity to it is called developing an energy sense. Because the pranic flow has been rejuvenated, a natural quieting and calming effect occurs in the mind. Allow yourself to drink in this opportunity for full body-mind ease. If you remain calmly alert yet free from engagement with any mental stimuli, you can experience a state of natural awareness, making this the most nourishing posture of all.

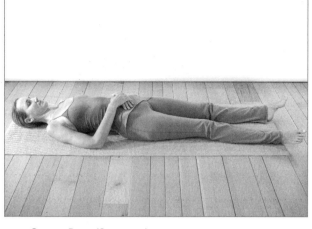

7.23. Corpse Pose (Savasana)

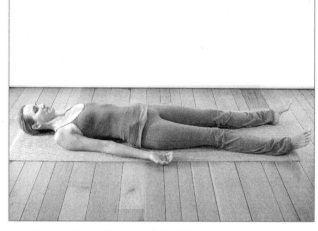

7.24. Corpse Pose (Savasana), Variation 1

Kidney/Urinary Bladder Long Session

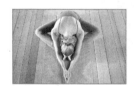 Butterfly Pose

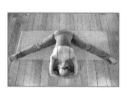 Dragonfly Pose

 Saddle Pose

 Lying Spinal Twist Pose (both sides)

 Sphinx Pose

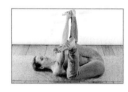 Stirrup Pose

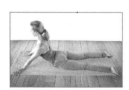 Seal Pose

 Legs-Up-the-Wall Pose

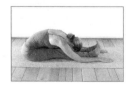 Full Forward Bend

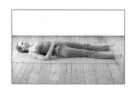 Corpse Pose (Savasana)

Follow the instructions given for the short session for Butterfly Pose (Fig. 7.25), Saddle Pose (Fig. 7.26), Sphinx Pose (Fig. 7.27), Seal Pose (Fig. 7.28), and Full Forward Bend (Fig. 7.29).

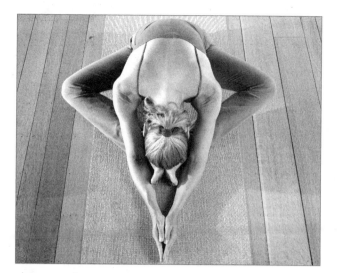

7.25. Butterfly Pose

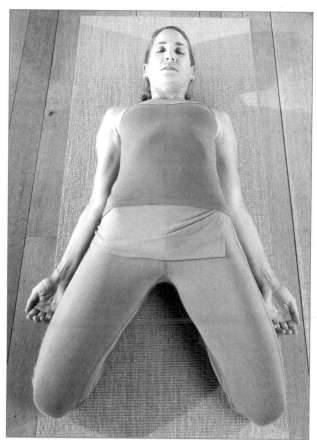

7.26. Saddle Pose

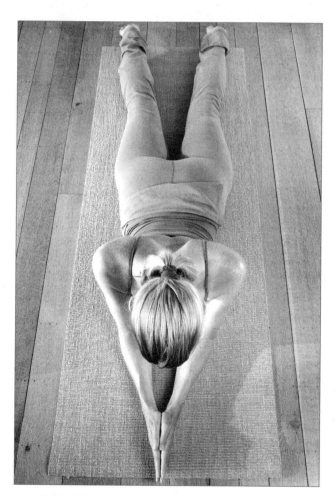

7.27. Sphinx Pose

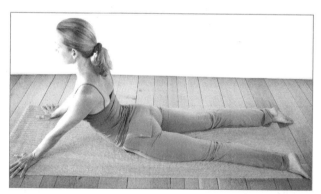

7.28. Seal Pose

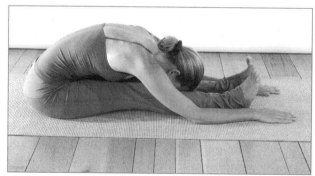

7.29. Full Forward Bend

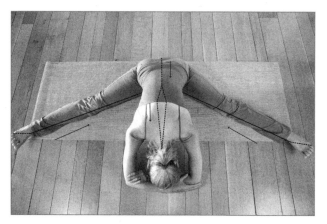

7.30. Dragonfly Pose—Kidney meridian shown

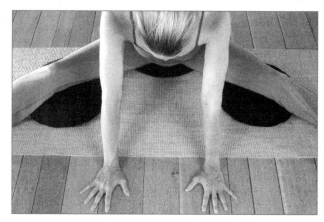

7.31. Dragonfly Pose, Variation 1

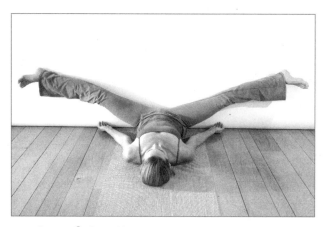

7.32. Dragonfly Pose, Variation 2

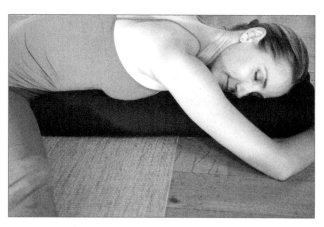

7.33. Dragonfly Pose, Variation 3

Dragonfly Pose

This pose stimulates the Kidney meridian as it flows along your inner legs, as well as the Bladder meridian as it flows down your back and the backs of your legs (Fig. 7.30).

Spread your legs as wide apart as they are willing to go. If they do not open very far, it may be more beneficial to bend your knees and place some padding under them to lessen the pull on the hamstrings. This will also allow you to fold forward from the hips a little better as it is easier to bend forward from the hips when the knees are bent rather than straight (Fig. 7.31).

Note: If you have tight hamstrings or are avoiding forward bends due to back issues or sciatica, you could also do this pose lying on your back with your legs up the wall (Fig. 7.32).

On an exhalation, shift the weight in your hips forward and begin to allow gravity to bring you down. If your knees are unstable, engage your quadriceps part of the time in this pose or any seated forward bend. Your hands can be on the floor in front of you, you can rest on your elbows, or you may support yourself on a cushion (Fig. 7.33).

Stay in this pose for 3 to 5 minutes. To come out, inhale and walk your hands back in, bringing your spine back to an upright position. Bring your legs together and rest back on your hands for a moment or two.

You may alternate this pose with Lateral Dragonfly Pose (described next) to emphasize the side body more.

Lateral Dragonfly Pose

Sit straight with your legs in a wide straddle. Shift forward on your sitting bones and lean to the left, placing your left elbow on the floor along the inside of your leg (or on a cushion) and allowing your head to rest in your left hand. Your right hand can stay at your side, or you can rest your right arm across your head, or reach for your left foot (Fig. 7.34). Hold this pose for 3 to 5 minutes, then release your left elbow and rotate your torso so you are resting facedown over your left leg with your arms extended and relaxed on either side of the leg (Fig. 7.35).

Stay in this pose for 3 to 5 minutes. To come out, inhale and raise up. Bring your body back to center for a few breaths before repeating on the other side.

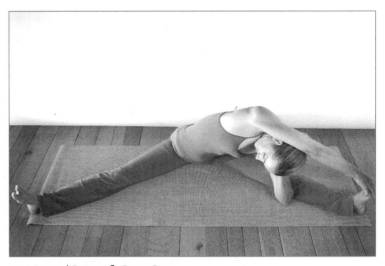

7.34. Lateral Dragonfly Pose, Part 1

Lying Spinal Twist Pose

This pose stimulates the Kidney and Bladder meridians along both sides of your spine, and the Kidney meridian along your inner legs and torso (Fig. 7.36).

Lie on your back with your knees bent, your feet flat on the floor, and your arms out to the sides for support. On an exhalation, allow your knees to drop to the left while keeping the right side of your upper back and shoulder weighted toward the floor. If your knees do not rest on the floor, use a bolster or folded blanket to catch their weight (Fig. 7.37). This is also a good suggestion if your lower back is sensitive or has been injured.

If you would like to emphasize drawing chi more toward your lower back, hug your knees closer toward your torso (Fig. 7.38). If you would like to target your hips and sacroileac region, then leave your knees in line with your hips or even a little lower (see Fig. 7.36).

Bring your right arm up to rest on the floor alongside your head (place a prop under your arm if it does not rest easily on the floor). This will encourage the energy distribution to pool in and around the shoulder area, another common place for chi stagnation. These tissues house the Lung,

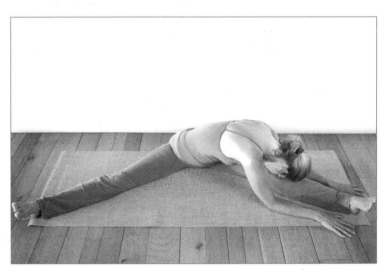

7.35. Lateral Dragonfly Pose, Part 2

Heart, and both Intestine meridians as well. If you would like to direct the impact more specifically into your right shoulder, turn your head away from your raised arm. If you want to feel it more along your upper back, look toward your raised arm.

You can alternate head positions as you hold the pose on each side. You can also look in one direction for half the time and turn your head the other way for the second half. Stay in the pose for 3 to 5 minutes.

To come out, first slide your right arm back down beside your torso on an exhale. Next, use an inhalation, your abdominal muscles, and your

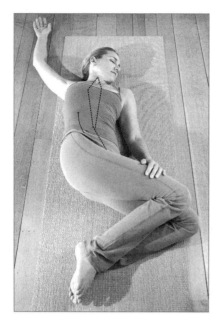

7.36. Lying Spinal Twist Pose—
Kidney meridian shown

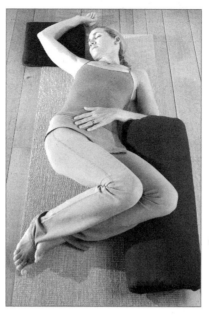

7.37. Lying Spinal Twist Pose, Variation 1

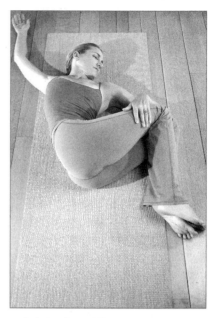

7.38. Lying Spinal Twist Pose, Variation 2

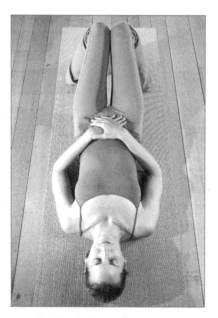

7.39. Resting in Neutral

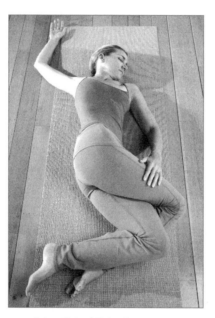

7.40. Lying Spinal Twist Pose, Variation 3

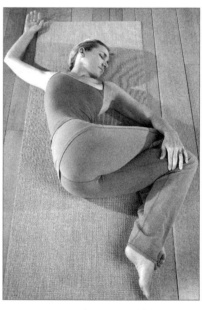

7.41. Lying Spinal Twist Pose, Variation 4

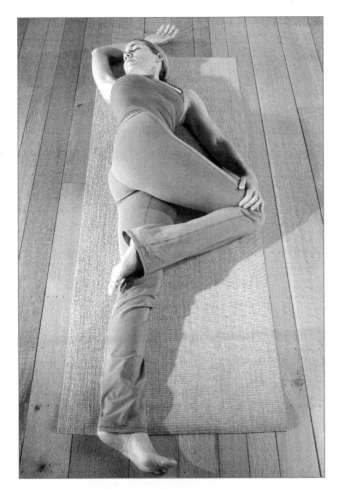

7.42. Lying Spinal Twist Pose, Variation 5

hands to bring your knees back up into a neutral position. Rest with your feet on the floor, and your knees dropping into each other (Fig. 7.39). Stay here for a few breaths before repeating the pose to the other side, with your knees dropping to the right and raising your left arm next to your head.

For an even deeper twist, you can cross one knee over the other (like when you're sitting with your legs crossed) before going over into the twist. In this crossed-knee variation, you may choose to rest your legs below hip-height to emphasize the pull in your hips (Fig. 7.40) or pull your knees in toward your ribs to strengthen the sensations in your lower back (Fig. 7.41).

You can also keep your left (bottom) leg straight and simply bend your right (top) knee as you twist to the left (Fig. 7.42). Hook your right foot behind your left leg as you twist, and once your weight is over on your left buttock, fold over to the right so your weight rests pre-

dominantly on your outer left hip. Remember that the farther your knees are from your torso, the greater the emphasis will be in your hips and sacral region; when your knees are closer to your ribs, the impact of chi distribution moves up your back.

This pose benefits all of your internal organs, which are gently massaged by the twisting motion. The Urinary and Gallbladder meridians, which run along the sides of your body, are also nourished in this pose.

Stirrup Pose

This pose stimulates the Kidney meridian (as well as the Liver and Spleen) as it flows up your inner legs (Fig. 7.43).

Lie on your back, bend your knees toward your chest, and reach your hands along your inner thighs to your feet. Place your hands on your inner arches and draw your feet out so they are positioned over your knees. You will look like you are squatting on the ceiling. Keep your chin in line with your forehead (if the head raises, place a cushion under it), your shoulders weighted toward the floor, and your sacrum down.

If you cannot hold your feet easily, place a strap around each foot and hold the ends of each strap in the corresponding hand. If you find the sensations in your groin or legs too intense, simply bring your feet down closer to your buttocks (Fig. 7.44).

You can also do this with your feet flat against a wall. Sit next to a wall with your right hip touching it. As you lie back, swivel around and take your feet up the wall; this should allow you to position your buttocks right up against the wall when you are lying flat with your legs above you. Bend your knees and plant your feet against the wall as low and wide as you can, as if you are squatting (Fig. 7.45). To come out, walk your feet back up the wall until the knees are straight. Rest here a few moments before bending the knees and rolling to the side, using your hands to sit up.

Stay in the pose for 3 to 5 minutes. To come out, exhale as you release your feet and draw your knees into your chest and clasp your hands over your lower legs for a few breaths or minutes (Fig. 7.46).

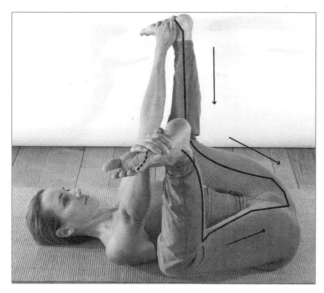

7.43. Stirrup Pose—Kidney meridian shown

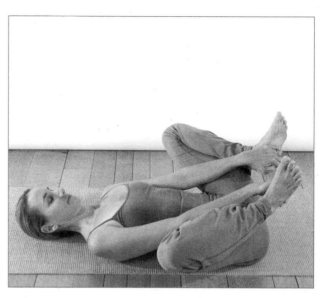

7.44. Stirrup Pose, Variation 1

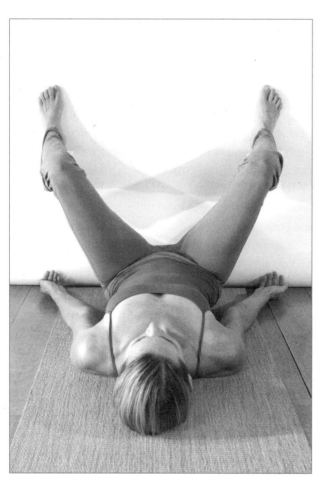

7.45. Stirrup Pose, Variation 2

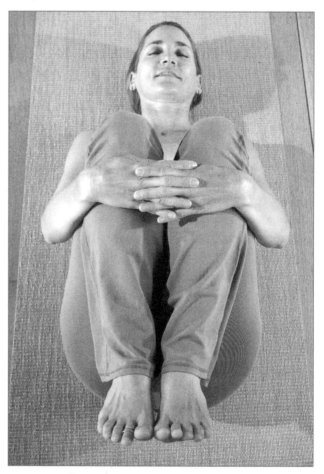

7.46. Knees-into-the-Chest Pose

Legs-Up-the-Wall Pose

This pose stimulates the Bladder meridian as it flows along the backs of your legs (Fig. 7.47). Complete instructions for this pose are given on page 46.

Corpse Pose (Savasana)

Full instructions for this pose (Fig. 7.48) are given on page 47.

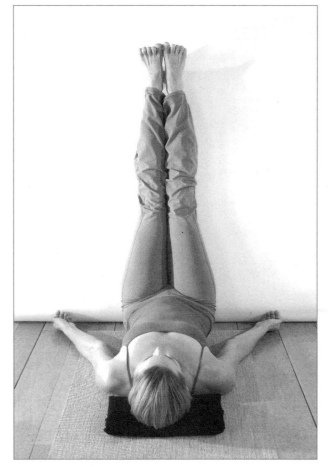

7.47. Legs-Up-the-Wall Pose

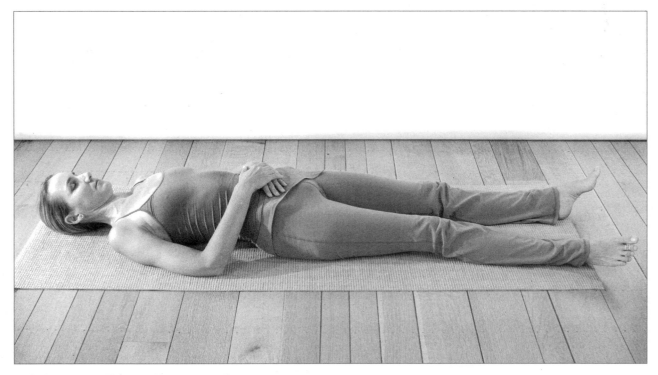

7.48. Corpse Pose (Savasana)

8

The Liver and Gallbladder

THE LIVER COMMANDED particular respect among the ancients, who considered it the seat of life, naming it the liver. The Old English word is *lifer*; in German it is *die Leber*, from the verb *leben*, meaning "to live."

Physical Qualities
Liver

The liver is the largest gland in the body, weighing three to four pounds. It lies on the right side of the abdominal cavity, just under the diaphragm, and is protected by the lower ribs. It is a major storage site for vitamins A, D, K, and B_{12}; minerals; and glycogen, which is converted to glucose as needed to provide energy. Insulin, a hormone produced by the pancreas, controls the amount of glucose in the blood. If the level is too high, it is called hyperglycemia (diabetes). When the level is too low, it is called hypoglycemia. The liver also stores the blood when we are at rest, releasing it for action when we move. When liver tissues are damaged, the active liver cells are replaced by fat cells and scar tissue. This is called cirrhosis of the liver, a chronic inflammation that leads to organ failure (often caused by alcoholism or an unknown etiology in infants). Hepatitus is a disease commonly caused by one of three viruses (A, B, or C), which progressively deteriorates the liver and can cause lifelong infection.

The liver is the primary chemical factory of the body. Any substance that cannot be broken down and used for energy ends up in the liver for detoxification. The liver continuously produces bile, a secretion that is stored in the gallbladder and is an important component for the digestion of foods. Bile is very concentrated, composed of several important elements, such as bile salts that assist in fat absorption. Without the proper amount of bile in our system, the fat we get from food would remain undigested, because enzymes from the pancreas only break down substances that can be dissolved in water, but oil-rich foods and animal products require the bile salts in order to be broken down.

Liver chi imbalances are linked to types of paralysis, arthritis, cramping, muscular weakness or stiffness, feeling off center, fatigue, vertigo, and dizziness, as well as dimmed vision, astigmatism, cataracts, and blindness. We can see by this list that healthy liver function is crucial.

Gallbladder

The gallbladder is a small sac into which the bile from the liver flows. Whereas the liver is considered the general of the army, the gallbladder is the upright official who is constantly making decisions for the entire body-mind. Its function is to store and secrete bile as an aid in the digestive process.

Energetic Qualities

As with the kidneys, the energetic functions connected with the liver far exceed its anatomical function. The Taoists thought healthy liver chi so central to our overall well-being that they nicknamed it "the general of the army." It is the military leader who excels at strategic planning, making sure the flow of energy within us happens harmoniously. Liver chi coordinates and regulates the movement of chi everywhere within us, which is responsible for creating an easygoing disposition and internal atmosphere.

Whereas kidney chi is responsible for a vibrant quality of inner energy, liver chi governs the overall healthy flow of energy. Liver chi also rules the health of the muscles, tendons, nails, hands, and feet. Its sense door is the eyes, which reflect the health of liver chi. Whereas the kidney is associated with the element of water, the liver is related more closely to wood, needing to be both stable and flexible, like a rooted tree. The liver chi is connected to our sense of sight and corresponds to the eyes. See the table on page 20 for more details.

Emotional Qualities

Since liver chi is responsible for an easygoing inner environment, it is also in charge of balancing the emotions. When we have a liver chi imbalance, we have a propensity for uneven, irregular emotions; chronic anger; explosive impulsivity; a defense of personal boundaries; and awkward social behavior. All aspects of resistance are connected with liver chi dysfunctions, from minor frustrations like annoyance and irritation to de-

fensiveness, divisiveness, or all-out rage. Whether we are on edge, ready to pick a fight at the slightest thing, or feeling paralyzed, stuck, and unable to express anger or defend ourselves, it is a call to attend to liver chi function. Whether there is a marked presence or complete absence of anger, this inner conflict is connected to liver chi disturbances. When we are chronically angry, we are stressing our liver chi; when liver chi is less functional, we find ourselves getting angry or easily upset. It works both ways.

A woman may notice during menstruation, for example, that she is a bit more irritable than usual. This is not only a result of hormonal influences and overreactivity in the limbic system, but also because her body is flushing out accumulated toxins, making the liver more active than at other times, affecting the liver chi. As a result, she may feel added discomfort in the Liver and Gallbladder meridians that run along the outer hips and inner legs. While in Yin poses, she may also experience an added level of frustration and annoyance for no apparent reason. This is a natural process that when understood, can reduce our resistance to feeling such inner tensions and allow us to move through them more graciously.

When we are experiencing liver chi imbalances, it is helpful to diminish our preoccupation with our irritations and gently turn toward our feelings. As we diminish acting out in a harsh way and increase sensitivity toward ourselves, we open pathways toward self-care, helping us stay attentive and connected to our bodies. This is the movement toward compassion, the emotion associated with liver chi harmony. For example, we can turn toward our foul mood with tenderness, while climbing into our body without any expectations of performance or comparisons of any kind. During these times, it is also helpful to practice metta and karuna meditational phrases while in Yin poses for the liver (see page 176 for more information on these phrases).

Mental Qualities

Liver chi is connected to our ability to make appropriate connections, a natural coordination of the mind. Healthy liver chi is related to a capacity to make plans and put them into action, exerting a sense of volitional control. Liver chi health is demonstrated by an ability to evaluate a situation and access the proper physical, emotional, and social conduct. The essential feature of liver chi health is flexibility and an ability to change and adapt. When there is a frustration in the system, it is hard to think, hard to plan. This chi disharmony is related to migraine headaches.

Liver/gallbladder chi is responsible for our discernment. The gallbladder relates to our ability to follow our path in life, to avoid deviating or being put off by external influences. It also relates to our capacity to regain equilibrium after a shock or obstructions in our plans. When we have an excess of liver/gallbladder chi, we tend to make rash decisions, and when the chi is depleted, we experience hesitation and timidity.

9

Yin Yoga Sequences for the Liver and Gallbladder

The Liver and Gallbladder Meridians

THE LIVER MERIDIAN begins at the top of the big toe and runs up along the inner leg, just above the Kidney meridian. It enters the torso through the groin, goes through the liver and gallbladder, into the lungs, and up through the throat into the head, circling the lips and moving into the eyes.

The Gallbladder meridian begins at the outer corner of the eye and travels down the lateral side of the body to the outer hip. An internal branch goes through the neck and chest into the liver and gallbladder. It runs down into the outer knee and ends in the fourth toe.

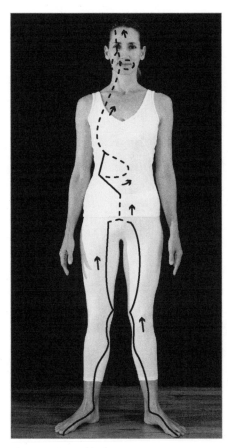

The Liver Meridian

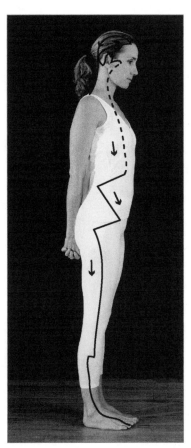

The Gallbladder Meridian

Liver/Gallbladder Short Session

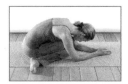 Shoelace Pose, or Eye-of-the-Needle Pose (both sides)

 Sphinx Pose, or Seal Pose

 Child's Pose

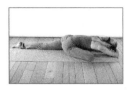 Sleeping Swan Pose, or Eye-of-the-Needle Pose

 Child's Pose

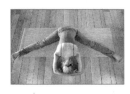 Dragonfly Pose

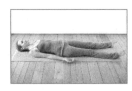 Corpse Pose (Savasana)

Shoelace Pose

The pressure this pose creates in the inner thighs stimulates the Liver meridian in the groin and pulls on the Gallbladder meridian as it travels down the outer hip and leg (Fig. 9.1).

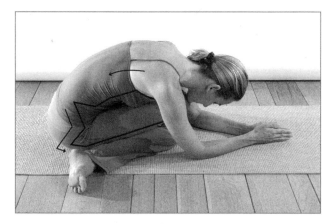

9.1. Shoelace Pose—Gallbladder meridian shown

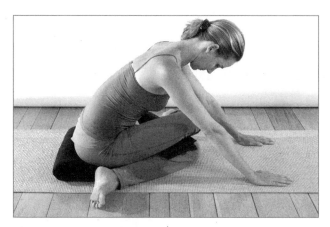

9.2. Shoelace Pose, Variation 1

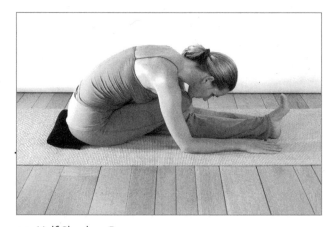

9.3. Half-Shoelace Pose

Begin by sitting straight with your right leg drawn over your left so that your knees are stacked and your feet are sitting back near your hips with your hands at your sides. If this external-hip-rotation range of motion is difficult for you, elevate your sitting bones on a cushion (Fig. 9.2). If there is space between your knees, put a folded blanket there as well.

If you have lower back sensitivity or knee weakness, you can avoid bending forward in this pose and simply sit up straight with your hands placed on the floor behind or in front of you. Another alternative is to stretch out your bottom leg to prevent too much pressure on your knees. This is called Half-Shoelace Pose (Fig. 9.3).

If this still feels risky in your top knee, you can take Eye-of-the-Needle Pose, which eliminates all gravitational pressure to your knees and is described next.

If you do decide to fold forward, remain vigilant about the kind of sensations you experience; make sure you feel this pose in your buttocks, outer hips, inner groin, or lower back rather than as a pull in your inner knees. You can rest your hands farther forward and round your back forward. Use the weight of your hands into the floor to distribute the impact of this pose to your hips instead of your knees. If you are all the way forward, push your elbows down as you come forward to keep your weight back in your hips and light on your knees.

If you feel limited by a thick feeling in your groin, allow your forward pressure to be slow and gradual, honoring the sensations of resistance by allowing your body weight to impose a slight pressure. Be patient and follow your body's feedback to determine if it is appropriate to go further.

Stay in this pose for 3 to 5 minutes.

To come out, inhale and, using your hands or abdominal muscles, lift your spine back up vertebra by vertebra, stretching your legs out in front of you and leaning back on your hands. Rest this way for a few breaths. Repeat with the left leg on top.

Eye-of-the-Needle Pose

Lie on your back with your feet on the floor and your knees bent; place your right ankle on top of your left knee. Draw your left knee toward your chest, reach your hands around your shin, and interlace your fingers (Fig. 9.4). Your left arm will reach around the outside of your left leg, and your right arm will reach between your legs. As you draw your knee toward you, keep your sacrum down, and your shoulders and head on the floor. If you cannot reach forward and clasp your hands easily, you can hold a strap between your hands, and/or place a small blanket under your head so that your chin and forehead rest at the same height.

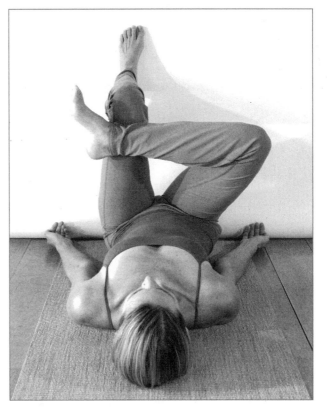

9.5. Eye-of-the-Needle Pose, Variation

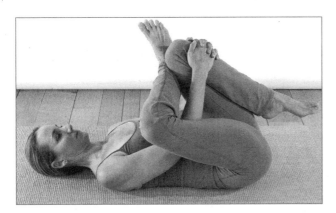

9.4. Eye-of-the-Needle Pose

Relax your left ankle and close your eyes while you remain in this pose for 3 to 5 minutes.

This pose can also be done if it is difficult to reach through and clasp your hands, with your left foot pressed against the wall and your right ankle crossed over your left knee, while your hands rest on the floor (Fig. 9.5). Repeat instructions for legs up the wall, and then allow your right ankle to rest over the left knee. Bend the left knee and place the left foot on the wall as far down as it can come without lifting the sacrum off the floor. Rest your hands on the floor or on your abdomen. To come out, take the right foot back up the wall and switch legs. After both sides have been held for 3 to 5 minutes, bend your knees and roll to your side, using your hands to sit up.

Seal Pose

Do Seal Pose (Fig. 9.7) as described on page 43.

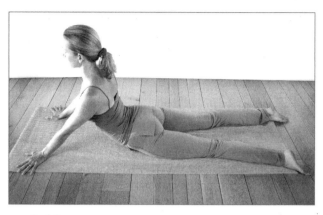

9.7. Seal Pose

Sphinx Pose

Do Sphinx Pose (Fig. 9.6) as described on page 41.

Child's Pose

Do Child's Pose (Fig. 9.8) as described on page 42.

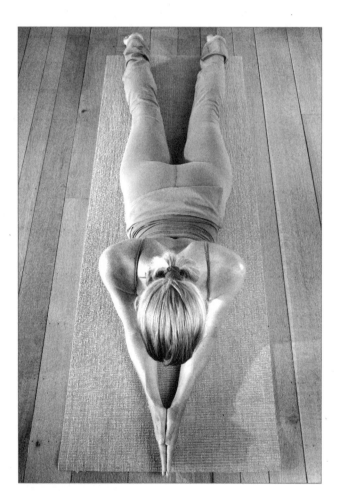

9.6. Sphinx Pose

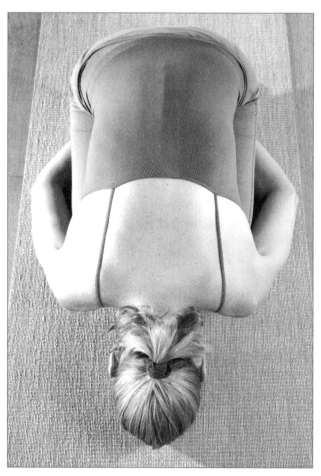

9.8. Child's Pose

Sleeping Swan Pose

This external rotation pose affects the Gallbladder meridian, which runs down the side of the body along the outer hip, and places pressure on the groin to nourish the Liver meridian (Fig. 9.9).

From Child's Pose, inhale and bring your right knee forward and place your shin and knee on the floor in front of and to the right of your right hip. If your right thigh does not rest on the floor or you have a sensitive knee, place a folded blanket or pillow under your right hip (Fig. 9.10).

Look back and make sure that your left leg is behind your left hip while allowing the left front hip to face the floor. You can rest your weight up on your hands for all or part of the time to prevent any stress to your knee (Fig. 9.11).

If you come down onto your forearms, push your elbows into the floor to shift your weight back into the hips. You can think of this pose as needing to be heavy in the hips and light on the front knee, *not* heavy in the knee and light in the hip.

If you still feel this pose is potentially risky to your right knee, then avoid it altogether and take Eye-of-the-Needle Pose instead (see page 63). Hold the pose for 3 to 5 minutes.

To come out, inhale up onto your hands. Exhale and draw your right foot behind your thigh. Rest back in Child's Pose. Repeat Sleeping Swan on the other side.

Dragonfly Pose

This pose affects theLiver meridian, which flows up the inner leg (Fig. 9.12). See page 50 for a complete description.

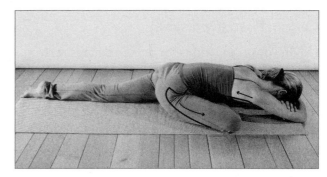
9.9. Sleeping Swan Pose—Gallbladder meridian shown

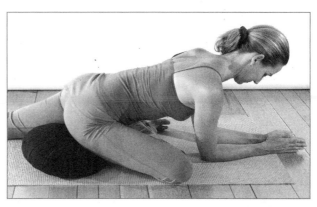
9.10. Sleeping Swan Pose, Variation 1

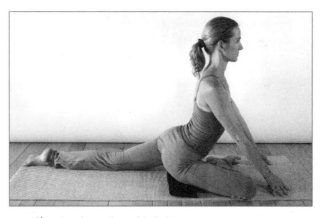
9.11. Sleeping Swan Pose, Variation 2

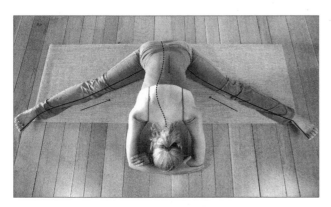
9.12. Dragonfly Pose—Liver meridian shown

Corpse Pose (Savasana)

Lie on your back with your arms and legs resting a few feet from center. Turn your palms up (Fig. 9.13), or place your hands lightly on your abdomen. Allow your feet to roll out or in as they like, and let your weight settle into the floor, resting your mind in your heart space.

Having pulled and pressured your tissues, it is now time to allow your body to rest fully, igniting the natural rescue remedy throughout your system. This organic psychophysical response within us flushes out unusable physical pollutants and mental distractions, while pulsing in rejuvenating energy and natural wakefulness. Bask in the natural ease of release that comes from having completed these restorative actions.

Rest in this pose 5 to 10 minutes.

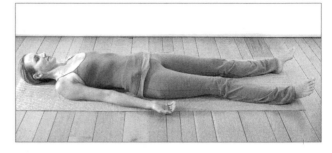

9.13. Corpse Pose (Savasana)

Liver/Gallbladder Long Session

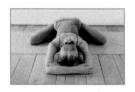 Wide-Knee Child's Pose

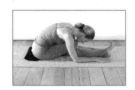 Half-Shoelace Pose

 Sphinx Pose, or Seal Pose

 Seated Twist Pose
(Now go back and repeat the other side, starting with Sleeping Swan Pose.)

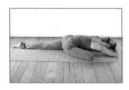 Sleeping Swan Pose

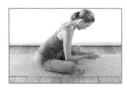 Square Pose
(both sides)

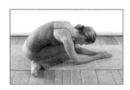 Shoelace Pose

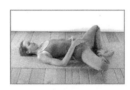 Lying Butterfly Pose

 Lateral Shoelace Pose
(both sides)

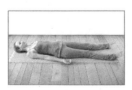 Corpse Pose (Savasana)

This sequence emphasizes external rotation in the hips to affect the Gallbladder and Liver meridians. It has you do a number of poses on one side to enhance the coaxing of chi on that side before moving on to the other. If this feels like too much sensation without relief, you can simply follow the list of poses suggested and do both right and left sides for each one. As these kinds of poses (external hip openers) tend to be more challenging for people, I have placed a Kidney pose close to the beginning (Seal Pose) and again near the middle (Half-Shoelace Pose) to restore your vitality along the way and assist you in persevering in the face of strong sensations and, at times, emotions.

Wide-Knee Child's Pose

Pulling the tissues in the inner thighs and groin during this pose (Fig. 9.14) affects the Liver channel.

From Child's Pose, spread your knees as wide as they are willing to go and keep your hips back in your arches. Rest forward on your forearms or chest, with your head either resting on your forearms or turned to one side. If you are protecting an injured groin area, be careful how far apart you spread your knees.

Stay in this pose for 3 to 5 minutes. To come out, bring your hands forward and on an inhale raise your hips away from the floor, then lift one knee and bring it toward the center of your body, following with the other knee. It is better not to drag your legs closer together after having been in this passive pose for so long.

Rest in Child's Pose.

Sphinx Pose

Do Sphinx Pose (Fig. 9.15) as described on page 41, or, if you can take a deeper backbend, do Seal Pose (Fig. 9.16) as described on page 43.

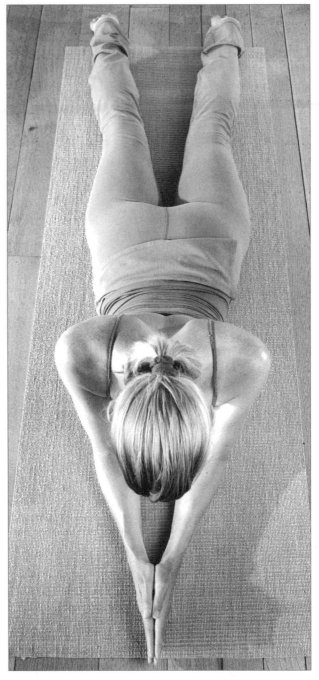

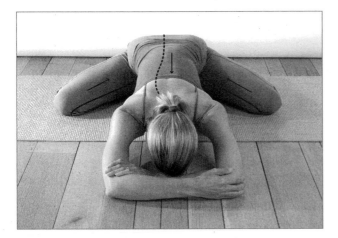

9.14. Wide-Knee Child's Pose—Liver meridian shown

9.15. Sphinx Pose

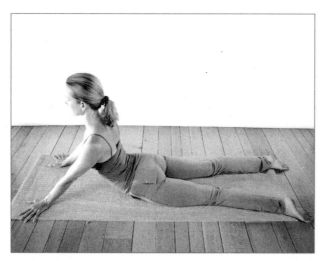

9.16. Seal Pose

Sleeping Swan Pose

Do Sleeping Swan Pose (Fig. 9.17) as described on page 65.

Shoelace Pose

Come up on your hands and bring the back leg forward, placing the right thigh on top in Shoelace Pose (Fig. 9.18). Follow the instructions on page 62 for this pose and its variations. Stay 3 to 5 minutes.

Lateral Shoelace Pose

Sitting with your right leg over your left, your knees stacked, put your weight on your right sitting bone. Allow your left hand to move out to the side, along the floor, in line with your left hip. If your right sitting bone stays on the floor and your hand is far out to the side, rest your forearm on the floor and drop your head to the left (Fig. 9.19).

Hold 2 to 3 minutes, return to center, for Half-Shoelace Pose.

Half-Shoelace Pose

This pose continues to nourish the Gallbladder meridian along the outer right hip, while adding emphasis to the Urinary Bladder meridian affected by the outstreched left leg (Fig. 9.20).

From Shoelace Pose (with a folded blanket still under your sitting bones so you can tilt forward from the hips), stretch your left leg out in front of you. If you have been feeling a lack of stability in

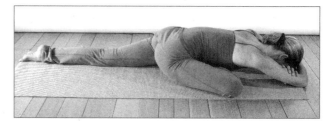
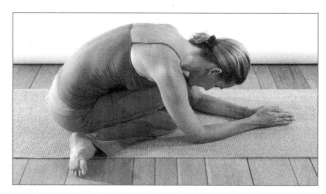

9.17. Sleeping Swan Pose

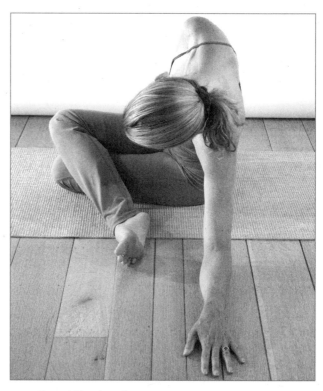

9.18 Shoelace Pose

9.19. Lateral Shoelace Pose

your left knee, you can keep your left quadricep engaged in this pose. If you have overstressed your hamstrings, then put a folded blanket under your left knee to avoid full extension. If your body does not come forward over your front leg at all due to tight hips and/or a tight lower back, then it is better to substitute Eye-of-the-Needle Pose for this one (see page 63).

Stay in this pose for 3 to 5 breaths. To come out, inhale and bring your torso upright.

Seated Twist Pose

This pose affects the Gallbladder meridian along the side of the hip, and the Liver meridian in the groin. (Fig. 9.21).

From Half-Shoelace Pose, bend your left knee and place your left foot near your right hip. Place your right foot on the floor outside your left knee (your right knee should be in the air), and bring your left hand or elbow around your right knee and rest your left hand on your left foot. Your right hand can be used as a prop on the floor behind you or placed on your inner left thigh. If this is awkward or risky for your left knee, extend your left leg out straight (Fig. 9.22). You can also try different placements for your left hand, such as on your right thigh (Fig. 9.23) or wrapped under your right knee, interlacing your fingers together (Fig. 9.24).

Unlike active twists in which you might continue to lift and twist breath to breath, here you simply place your body in the shape, allowing your chest to be lifted, while breathing slowly into the pose. Take slow, conscious breaths as your diaphragm will act as an inner massage as it passes by your digestive organs.

Stay in this pose for 3 to 5 minutes. To come out, exhale and release your left arm, bringing your right foot back next to the left, so you can rest in Child's Pose.

From Child's Pose, come forward with your left knee and repeat the sequence beginning with Sleeping Swan Pose on the left side. As before, follow it with Shoelace Pose, Lateral Shoelace Pose, Half-Shoelace Pose, Seated Twist Pose, and then Child's Pose.

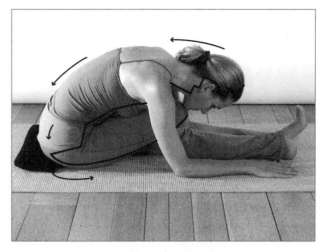

9.20. Half-Shoelace Pose—Gall Bladder Meridian Shown

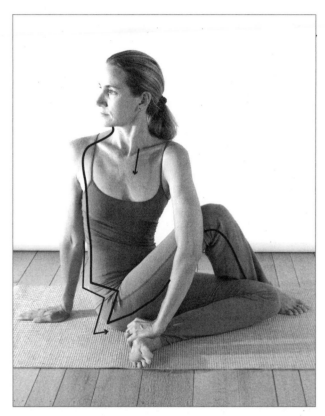

9.21. Seated Twist Pose—Gallbladder meridian shown

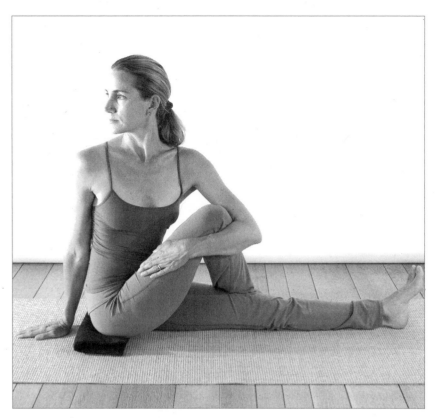

9.22. Seated Twist Pose, Variation 1

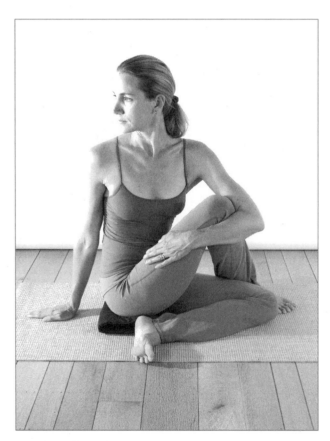

9.23. Seated Twist Pose, Variation 2

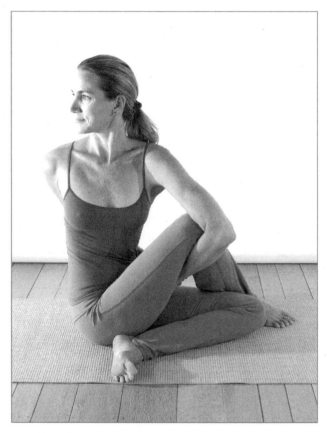

9.24. Seated Twist Pose, Variation 3

Square Pose

This pose affects the Gallbladder meridian along your outer hips and places pressure on the Liver channel in your inner groin (Fig. 9.25).

Sit cross-legged and bring your right foot on top of your left knee, your left foot under your right knee, your shins one on top of the other. You can place a cushion under your sitting bones to help the forward tilt of the pelvis. When you look down, you should see a triangle shape between your legs. If your right knee is not resting on your left foot, place a blanket under your right thigh and under your sitting bones (Fig. 9.26).

If this pose places too much pressure on your left knee, simply place your right foot on the outside of the knee on the floor in a simple seated cross-legged pose (Fig. 9.27). If seated forward bends do not aggravate your lower back, lean your weight forward at the hips and place your forearms on your shins, or your forearms on the floor in front of your shins (Fig. 9.28).

Stay in this pose for 3 to 5 minutes. To come out, inhale and bring your spine to an upright position and while leaning back, stretch out your legs, resting back on your hands before repeating the same pose on the other side.

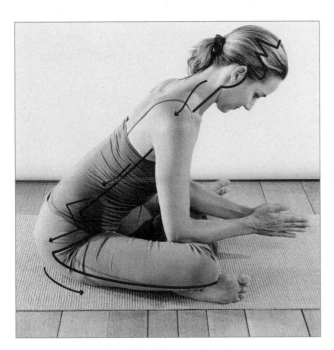

9.25. Square Pose—Gallbladder meridian shown

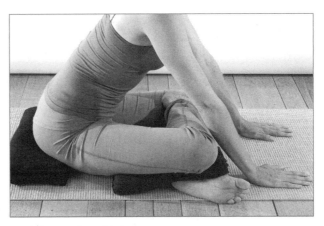

9.26. Square Pose, Variation 1

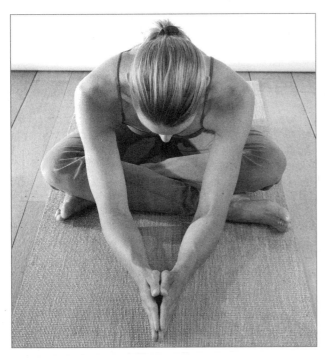

9.27. Square Pose, Variation 3

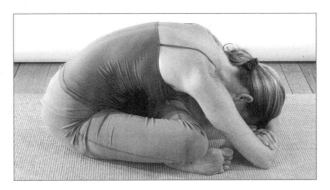

9.28. Square Pose, Variation 2

Lying Butterfly Pose

Do Lying Butterfly Pose (Fig. 9.29) as described on page 39.

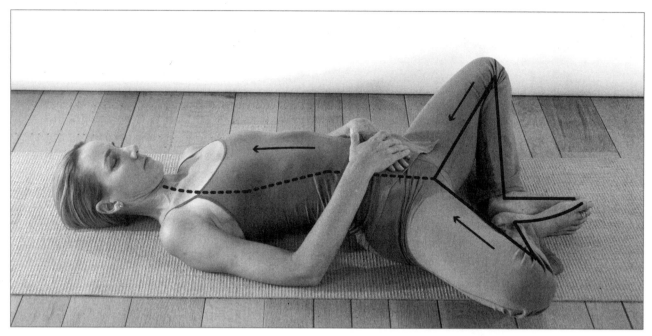

9.29. Lying Butterfly Pose—Liver meridian shown

Corpse Pose (Savasana)

Do Corpse Pose (Savasana; Fig. 9.30) as described on page 47.

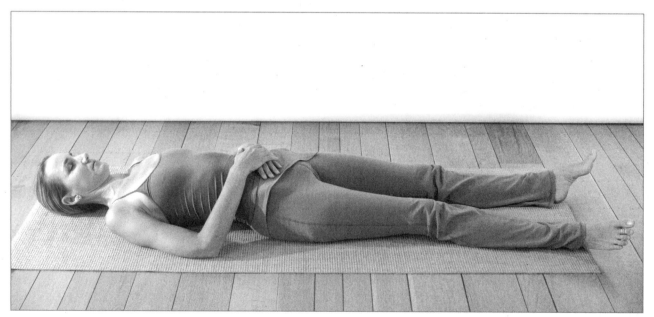

9.30. Corpse Pose (Savasana)

10

The Spleen and Stomach

THE SPLEEN AND STOMACH are the two organs most affected by our diet. As is true with the other organ-meridian pairs, the spleen and stomach have different physical functions but similar energetic, mental, and emotional characteristics. As with the gallbladder, we can live without our spleen, but the spleen's (or gallbladder's) energetic functions course through the meridians and continue to influence our nature, even if the organ has been removed.

Physical Qualities

Spleen

The spleen is a primary organ of digestion, a blood reservoir (supplying the body with blood in emergencies), and about the same size as the heart. It sits just behind the stomach on the left side, under the diaphragm. It produces lymphocytes, which destroy and recycle old red blood cells. The spleen is also the site where white blood cells, which fight infection, trap organisms.

Stomach

The stomach lies to the left of the diaphragm, between the esophagus and the intestines. It is the primary organ of digestion, receiving food and beginning the process of assimilation and distribution. The usable nutrients are sent to the spleen and the impure aspects to the small intestine for further filtration. Food usually stays in the stomach three to four hours before passing on. The stomach provides one of the most valuable functions of all because our energy is nourished by it on all levels, whether for physical, mental, or psychic growth. Taking in unpolluted food (appropriate for our constitution) and water is extremely important for healthy functioning, as the main disruption to healthy stomach chi is our diet.

Energetic Qualities

The spleen is thought of as the source of life for other organs because it extracts the pure nutritive essences of ingested food and liquids and converts them into blood and chi. It sends this "grain chi" upward in a mist to the lungs, where the synthesis of blood and chi take place. When spleen chi is out of balance, the whole system can become disharmonious, causing the whole body to develop impaired chi or impure blood.

When spleen chi is balanced, our cycles are in harmony. This allows all aspects of our life to be absorbed for psychosomatic nourishment. We feel earthy, sensual, full. When spleen chi is out of balance, the whole body-mind will not receive enough usable energy, causing lethargy, weakness, or dullness. Our rhythms, such as sleeping, breathing, and thinking, will be off. Ulcers, anorexia, obesity, infertility, or feelings of being ungrounded are all signs of spleen chi depletion. Spleen/stomach chi is connected to our sense of touch and secretion of saliva and corresponds to the mouth.

Emotional Qualities

Spleen chi is connected with the earth element and a sense of being at home inside ourselves. It is related to the ability to take in nourishment on all levels of the body-mind-spirit. Spleen chi is the link between the self and the world outside, transforming broccoli and carrots into us. This quality of adaptation is connected psychologically with spontaneity, our ability to assess a situation and come up with an appropriate response. Spleen chi is associated with our connection to the world around us, a relational capacity growing out of a sense of contentment, an ability to be at ease wherever we are.

Imbalanced spleen chi is associated with feelings of anxiety, nervousness, worry, pensiveness, sympathy-craving, and off-centeredness. These chronic emotions can also produce irritations and sores in the mouth, the sense door of spleen chi.

Mental Qualities

Spleen chi is associated with clear thinking, a capacity to make connections and garner understanding and insight. It is related to a sense of coherence, when various perceptions and ideas come together in a meaningful way that fosters accomplishment. Disharmonious spleen chi is connected with dogmatic thinking, obsessiveness, and inflexibility.

II

Yin Yoga Sequences for the Spleen and Stomach Organ-Meridians

Spleen and Stomach Meridians

THE SPLEEN MERIDIAN begins at the medial side of the big toe and comes up the inside of the leg, just next to the Liver channel. It goes into the torso through the groin; enters the stomach and spleen; goes up through the diaphragm, chest, and heart; and ends at the root of the tongue.

The Stomach meridian begins next to the nose and goes down through the diaphragm, into the stomach and spleen, moves down along the top of the leg, and ends at the second toe.

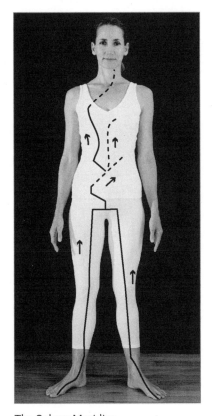

The Spleen Meridian

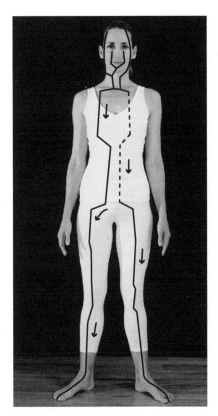

The Stomach Meridian

Spleen/Stomach Short Session

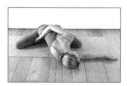
Wide-Knee Child's Pose with Twist

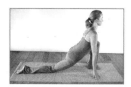
Dragon Pose (both sides)

Saddle Pose, or Sphinx Pose

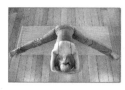
Dragonfly Pose

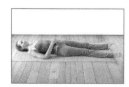
Corpse Pose (Savasana)

Wide-Knee Child's Pose with Twist

This pose affects the Spleen meridian along your inner legs, and the Stomach channels that flow down the front of your belly are nourished by the twisting (Fig. 11.1).

Begin in Child's Pose, then spread your knees as wide as they are willing to go, keeping your hips back near your feet. Twist to the left and take your right shoulder toward your left knee; rest it on the floor with your arm outstretched. Your left hand can reach around and rest on your lower back, or come around to your inner right thigh. Rest your head on the floor or your upper right arm.

Stay in this pose for 3 to 5 minutes. To come

out, release the left hand down on an exhale, and as you push into the floor to come up, slide your weight over to the other side, moving the left arm over to the right, resting on the left shoulder and taking your right arm back. Stay 3 to 5 minutes. To come out, exhale as you bring the right hand back to the floor. Inhale as you come up, pushing down through the right hand. With your weight on both hands, bring the knees back together, resting in Child's Pose. It is better not to drag your legs closer together after having been in this passive pose for so long. Simply lift one knee and bring it toward the center of your body, following with the other knee.

Rest in Child's Pose for a few breaths.

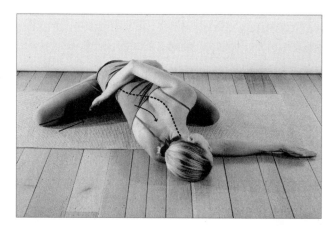
11.1. Wide-Knee Child's Pose with Twist—Spleen meridian shown

Dragon Pose

From Child's Pose, push up on all fours and step your left foot forward into a lunge. Allow your hips to draw forward toward your left foot until you feel an appropriate amount of intensity along the inner top of the right leg. You can rest your hands or fingertips on the floor (Fig. 11.2) or on blocks on either side of your left foot, allowing your right leg to be extended far back behind you.

You can also place your hands or elbows on the inside of your front leg (Fig. 11.3), which is especially helpful if you are pregnant.

Stay in this pose for 3 to 5 minutes. To come out, simply bring your weight back, away from your left foot, and exhale as you bring the left knee in line with the right. To change sides, come forward with your right foot and repeat on this side

11.2. Dragon Pose—Stomach meridian shown

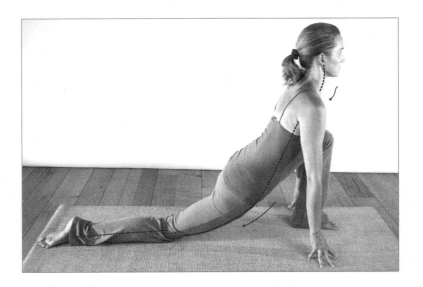

11.3. Dragon Pose, Variation

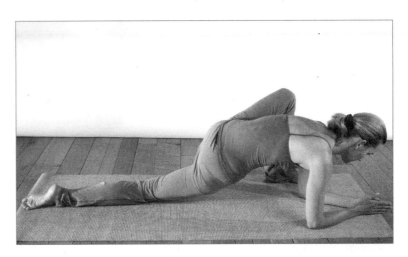

for 3 to 5 minutes. To come out, bring the right knee back in line with the left and rest back in Child's Pose.

Saddle Pose

Do Saddle Pose (Fig. 11.4) as described on page 39. As our main interest is emphasizing the top of the thighs where the stomach meridian flows, you can try placing your feet beside your hips in Saddle Pose, rather than keeping them under you. If this pose is risky for your knees, take Sphinx Pose as described on page 67 (Fig. 9.15).

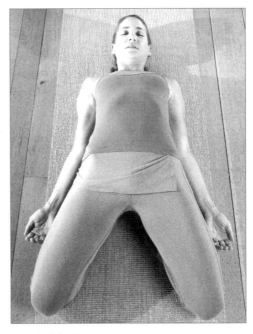

11.4. Saddle Pose

Dragonfly Pose

Dragonfly stimulates the Spleen meridian as it flows up the inner thighs. Do Dragonfly Pose (Fig. 11.5) as described on page 50.

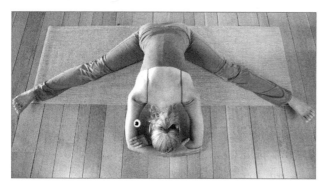

11.5. Dragonfly Pose—Spleen meridian shown

Corpse Pose (Savasana)

Do Corpse Pose (Savasana; Fig. 11.6) as described on page 47.

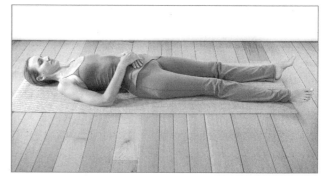

11.6. Corpse Pose (Savasana)

Spleen/Stomach Long Session

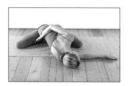 Wide-Knee Child's Pose with twist

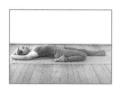 Half-Saddle Pose

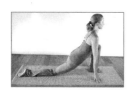 Dragon Pose

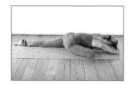 Sleeping Swan Pose (with left knee forward first)

 Child's Pose
(Repeat the sequence starting with Half-Saddle Pose with the left knee folded back.)

 Saddle Pose

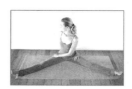 Dragonfly Pose with Twist

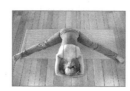 Dragonfly Pose, or Butterfly Pose

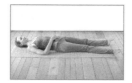 Corpse Pose (Savasana)

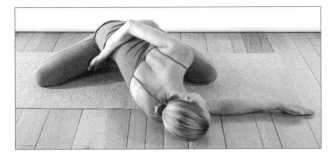

11.7. Wide-Knee Child's Pose with Twist

Wide-Knee Child's Pose with Twist

Do Wide-Knee Child's Pose (Fig. 11.7) as described on page 76.

Half-Saddle Pose

This pose stimulates the Stomach meridian as it flows down the top of the thigh (Fig.11.8).

From Child's Pose, sit up while leaning to your right side and stretch out your left leg, allowing your right leg to stay folded back with the foot near your buttocks. Rest back on your hands or elbows, or all the way back onto the floor. If you would prefer to put a little less flexion in your right knee, place some padding under your buttocks and behind your right knee (Fig. 11.9). You can also have support under your back and head.

Stay in this pose for 3 to 5 minutes.

To come out, inhale and lift up using your elbows and then your hands; engage your abdominals to help you move up out of the pose. Come into Dragon with your left foot forward.

When you would like to create variations with this practice, you can add a few poses from Half-Saddle Pose, before you come forward into Dragon. Simply come up from the backbend and, keeping your right leg still folded back, spread your knees wide and fold toward the left leg (Fig. 11.10). Hold for 3 to 5 minutes. Inhale, come up, and keeping your legs the same as the last pose, bring your torso centered between the legs and fold forward (Fig. 11.11). Stay here 3 to 5 minutes. Finally, still with your right leg folded back and your knees still wide, twist toward the right and reach your left hand to the outside of the right leg and your right hand can reach for the inner left leg, or rest on the floor behind you (Fig. 11.12).

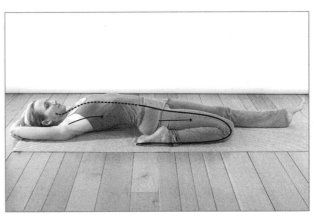

11.8. Half-Saddle Pose—Stomach meridian shown

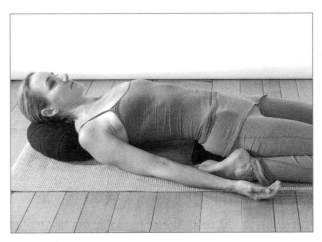

11.9. Half-Saddle Pose, Variation 1

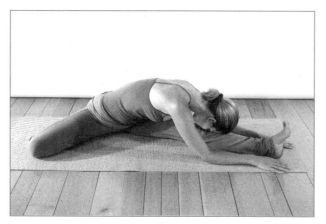

11.10. Half-Saddle Pose, Variation 2

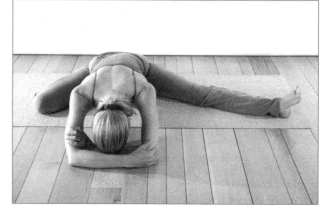

11.11. Half-Saddle Pose, Variation 3

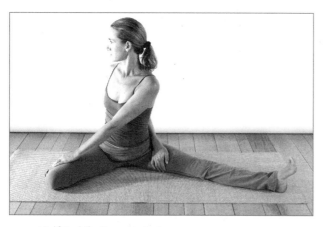

11.12. Half-Saddle Pose, Variation 4

Dragon Pose

Do Dragon Pose (Fig. 11.13) by lifting up out of Half-Saddle Pose and bending your left knee. Step your weight forward, into a lunge with the left foot forward, stretching the right leg back. (Note: this will relieve the right knee from the flexion of Half-Saddle.)

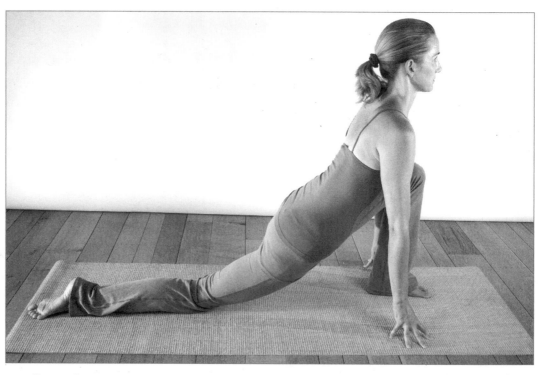

11.13. Dragon Pose

Sleeping Swan Pose

This pose stimulates the Spleen meridian—the groin of the front leg and along the inner thigh of the back leg (Fig.11.14).

From Dragon Pose, walk your left foot to the right and place your shin and knee on the floor in Sleeping Swan Pose. (Note the photo shows the right leg, but you are doing the left side first in this sequence.) Bring your left knee over to the left so the left foot rests in line with the center of your body. See page 65 for further instructions.

Stay in this pose for 3 to 5 minutes.

To come out, inhale and lift your hips while sliding your left foot under your left hip and going back to Child's Pose.

Repeat the same sequence on the other side with the left foot folded back in Half-Saddle Pose and then the right foot forward in Dragon Pose and Sleeping Swan. When you come out, rest in Child's Pose for a few breaths.

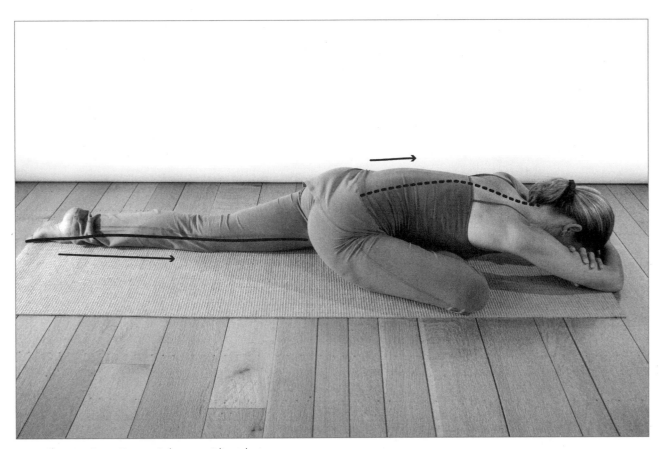

11.14. Sleeping Swan Pose—Spleen meridian shown

Saddle Pose

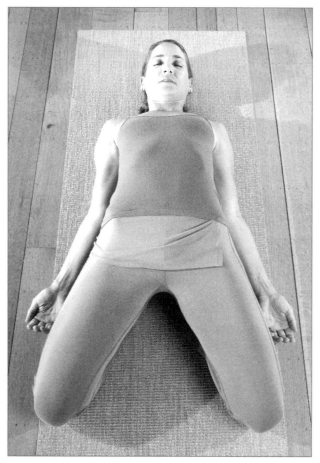

11.15. Saddle Pose

This pose stimulates the Spleen meridian along the inner leg and both the Spleen and Stomach meridians as they flow along the abdomen (Fig. 11.16).

Begin by sitting upright with your legs out in front of you. Then spread your legs as wide apart as they are willing to go in a straddle. If they do not pull open very far, it may be more beneficial to bend your knees and put the feet flat on the floor before bending forward. Take your right hand behind you toward your left thigh, and the left hand over to the outside of your right leg. If your right hand cannot reach all the way around, place it on the floor behind you. Keep your spine upright between your hips as you twist toward the right. Turn your head either toward the right or all the way to the left, or alternate.

Stay in this pose for 3 to 5 minutes. To come out, exhale, release the hands, and bring your body back to center. Repeat the twist toward the other side.

Dragonfly Pose

Do Dragonfly Pose (Fig. 11.17) as described on page 50. Or choose Butterfly Pose (Fig. 11.18), as described on page 38.

Do Saddle Pose (Fig. 11.15) as described on page 39.

Dragonfly Pose with Twist

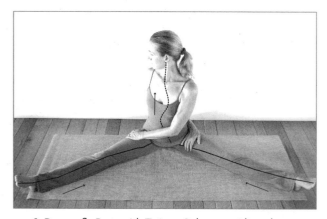

11.16. Dragonfly Pose with Twist—Spleen meridian shown

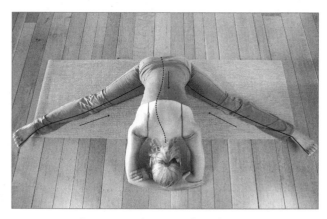

11.17. Dragonfly Pose—Spleen meridian shown

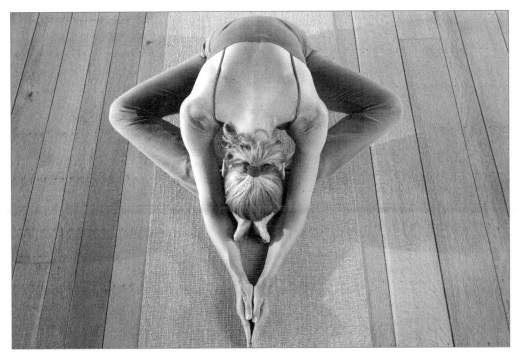

11.18. Butterfly Pose

Corpse Pose (Savasana)

Do Corpse Pose (Savasana; Fig. 11.19) as
described on page 47.

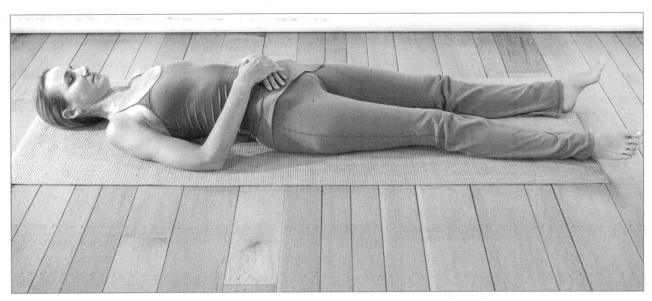

11.19. Corpse Pose (Savasana)

12

The Lungs and Large Intestine

THE LUNGS HOLD THE PRIVILEGE of being the life-giving network of the whole body, and all our functions depend on them for sustenance. Although they are not physically connected to the intestines, they share energetic characteristics that link them into an ongoing cycle of drawing in nutrients and letting go of waste.

Physical Qualities

Lungs

The lungs are vastly complex sponges that extend from the collarbones to the diaphragm, filling almost the entire chest cavity. The right lung is divided into three lobes, but the left has only two (because of the position of the heart). The lungs do a vital job: each day we take about twenty-three thousand breaths, which are filtered through our lungs to add fresh oxygen to our blood, which in turn carries that oxygen to each and every cell. We expel carbon dioxide (a waste gas from the metabolism of food) from our blood through our lungs as we exhale. They are a vast network that takes in, filters, assimilates, utilizes, and discards.

The Large Intestine

The large intestine is about five feet long and includes the colon and rectum. It is where we store and eliminate waste. It is the garbage collector and is responsible for absorption of water and excretion of solid waste material. When waste builds up, the rest of the system takes on a load it is not meant to bear, and this can result in diarrhea or constipation, bad acne, or headaches.

Energetic Qualities

The lungs are considered one of the most tender organs because they are the first area to assimilate the chi from the outside with the chi on the inside. They are the main way we replenish our energy and help organic processes to function within us. The lungs are considered the officials who receive the pure chi from the heavens on an inhalation and propel it downward to where kidney energy roots it in. If we catch a lot of colds or frequently feel under the weather, our lung chi (which is connected with our protective chi) is definitely weak. The nose and throat are also closely related to the lungs, as they are the thoroughfare for respiration. When lung chi is deficient, there can be deficient or stagnant chi anywhere in the body. This is reflected in an inability to take in on many levels, with symptoms ranging from allergies to asthma, bronchitis, respiratory disorders, shortness of breath, coughing and wheezing, rashes, or hives. Other problems that may arise when lung chi is poor are rheumatic pain, degeneration of the spine, and spasms of the throat and esophagus. These problems are associated with a breakdown within the network that keeps all the systems communicating. The skin is considered the "third lung" and relates to issues regarding acne, rashes, and hives (also connected with spleen chi). The element related to the lung is metal, as metals comprise our communication systems. Just as minerals of the earth provide nourishment for the soil, and as most structures rely on metal for reinforcement, lung chi nourishes and bolsters every cell of the body. Metals conduct electricity just as the breath conducts chi. Lung chi is connected to our sense of smell and corresponds to the nose.

Emotional Qualities

The lung–large-intestine chi is associated with courage and reverence, with an ability to experience our moments as precious and to stay in the experience we're in. Reverence is poignancy without the feeling of despair. It's what causes us to cry when we are awed by beauty. An imbalance or depletion in lung chi is linked to grief that is associated with loss. All emotions associated with the organs are considered natural responses to life. Yet when they become compulsive or prolonged, they become injurious to our overall health. Poor lung chi is expressed not only through extended bouts of sadness, but also by feeling emotionally stopped up or unable to express grief.

Mental Qualities

Healthy lung–large-intestine chi is connected with an ability to encounter difficulty with tenacity, a willingness to endure, and personal confidence. When lung chi is deficient, our thinking is muddled, cloudy, and disconnected.

13

The Heart and Small Intestine

T HE HEART'S RADIANCE spreads out to every cell and expresses itself in our creativity, interactions, and capacity for communication. Like the connection between the lungs and large intestine, the heart and small intestine are physically distant in the body and serve different physical functions, but energetically they resonate with the same characteristics.

Physical Qualities

The Heart

The heart lies in the chest cavity between the lungs and is a large muscle that is neither skeletal nor visceral. It is called a cardiac muscle because it has the strength and force of contraction of skeletal muscles but the involuntary control of visceral organs. It is the size of a human fist and is centrally located with a point that juts out to the left. It is responsible for supplying the body with oxygenated blood.

The Small Intestine

The small intestine is coiled in the center of the abdominal cavity and is where the most extensive part of digestion takes place. It receives what the stomach has not completely decomposed and continues the process of separation and absorption. This is the place where we sort out what's important from what's discardable on all levels in both body and mind. Hemorrhoids, abdominal pain, diarrhea, and constipation are related to excess heat in the system caused by an imbalance in the fire element.

Energetic Qualities

The heart–small-intestine chi's primary function is to rule the blood. Chi forms a yin/yang pair with blood. The concept of blood in Chinese medicine is quite different from the Western concept of blood. Blood is considered the yin aspect of chi; it is the aspect responsible for receptivity rather than engagement. Whereas chi is active, blood gives us the capacity to embrace and be comfortable with what has already been created. Chi gives us the ability to respond; blood gives us the ability to be comfortable being still.

The heart is considered the supreme manager, overseeing all the workings of the body-mind. It directs energy and is inextricably linked with the life principle, as its rhythm is our life giver. When heart–small-intestine chi is balanced, we are active, alive, full of vitality. When it is out of balance, we experience poor circulation, hardening of the arteries, cold hands and feet, hot flashes, heartburn, digestive problems, varicose veins, hemorrhoids, or heart disease. The heart and small intestine are related to the element of fire, actively sweeping through every area of our life. Heart chi is connected to our sense of taste and corresponds with the tongue.

Emotional Qualities

The heart chi is considered the monarch that looks after the whole kingdom:

> According to chapter eight of the *Ling Shu*, the liver often works with the heart to generate emotions because "that which goes hither and thither with the spirit is called the soul (*hun*)." Since the soul is stored in the liver and the spirit is stored in the heart, these two organs work together in the process of creating disordered emotional states.
>
> —*Yong Ping Jiang, DOM, PhD*

When the heart chi is healthy, we feel warm, nourished, and nourishing, able to contact innate joy, inner peace, and harmony, and able to build healthy relationships. Heart chi is related to to our vital center and spiritedness, and when it is out of balance, there may be a propensity for acute sadness, desperation, joylessness, depression, and estrangement when depleted, or cold intolerance, cruelty, and hatred when in excess. When the small intestine chi is out of balance, there is poor sorting, and unclear information and emotions dominate and deteriorate the inner system. When the heart–small intestine chi is harmonious, we have access to our intrinsic happiness and are able to bear witness to and intimately relate with all sides of life, whether we find ourselves in Hades or Heaven.

Mental Qualities

Healthy heart chi is related to a broad intelligence and connection with life, an understanding of its interconnectedness. Healthy heart–small-intestine chi allows us to experience the basic meaningfulness of life and to remain versatile and purposeful as we move through many changes. When it's out of balance, our sense of bonding is obscured by depression or hatred for circumstances and people.

14

Yin Yoga Session for the Lung, Heart, and Intestines Organ-Meridian Pairs

Lung, Heart, and Small and Large Intestine Meridians

THE LUNG MERIDIAN begins in the middle of the body and runs down into the large intestine before it makes a turn upward, moving through the diaphragm, into the lungs, across the front of the

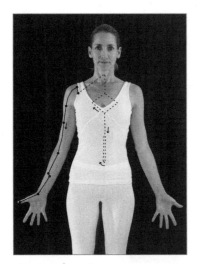

The Lung Meridian

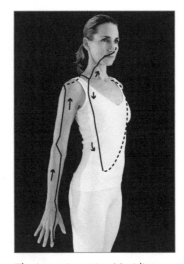

The Large Intestine Meridian

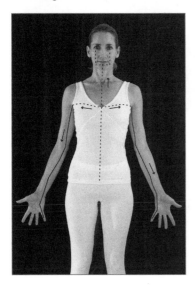

The Heart Meridian

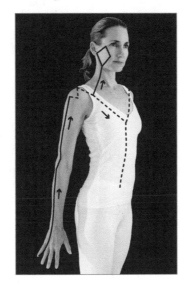

The Small Intestine Meridian

clavicle and down the inner arm, ending at the tip of the thumb.

The Large Intestine meridian begins at the tip of the index finger and goes up the back of the arm to the shoulder, where one branch goes through the neck and mouth to the side of the nose and another branch goes down into the lungs, diaphragm, and large intestine.

The Heart meridian has three branches, each of which begins in the heart. One runs down through the diaphragm to the small intestine. Another runs up through the throat and tongue to meet the eye. The third runs across the chest and down the inner arm, ending at the tip of the little finger.

The Small Intestine meridian begins in the little finger and runs up the outer arm to the shoulder, where it splits into two branches. One runs down into the heart, diaphragm, stomach, and small intestine; the other runs up into the face and across the corner of the eye to the ear.

The following four meridians are outside the scope of this book, but I have explained them here so you have a complete list of the fourteen major meridians. Please see the Suggested Readings at the back of this book for further information.

The Pericardium, Triple Heater, Conception Vessel, and Governor Vessel

The pericardium is a sac that surrounds the heart, which is where the corresponding meridian begins. One branch goes down into the diaphragm

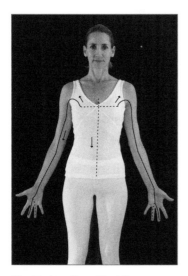

The Pericardium Meridian

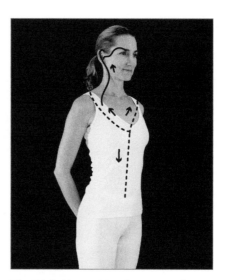

The Triple Heater Meridian

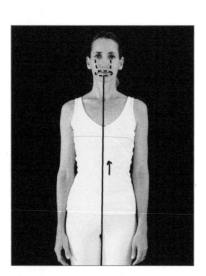

The Conception Vessel

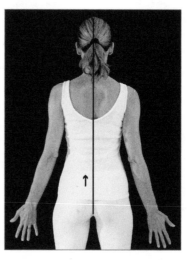

The Governor Vessel

and lower belly a few inches below the navel. Another branch runs down the inner arm to end at the tip of the middle finger. It guides love and intimate relationships, circulation, the hormones, and sexual functions, causing it to also be called the "circulation sex" meridian. Chinese medicine suggests that there are hundreds of symptoms connected with the function of the pericardium that usually go undiagnosed in Western medicine. Along with the Triple Heater it is thought to be one of the great gifts of Chinese Medicine.

The Triple Heater meridian begins in the ring finger and travels up the arm over the shoulder, where it splits into two branches. One branch goes through the pericardium and diaphragm, making its way down a few inches below the navel. Another branch goes up the neck, around the ear and head, encircling the face. Although there is no anatomical correlate, the Triple Heater is thought to control all internal heat functions and maintain the functioning of all the organs. The Triple Heater relates to three areas in the body, sometimes called three burning spaces: the upper, middle, and lower. The upper is the heart and lungs, connected with respiration and circulation. The middle is the stomach, spleen, gallbladder, liver, pancreas, and small intestine, all related with digestion. The lower is the large intestine, bladder, and kidneys, related with elimination. When the Triple Heater has gone askew, it can cause all kinds of physical and emotional disturbances as it distributes yang fire energy to all the inner organs.

The Conception Vessel meridian originates in the pelvis at the perineum, flowing up the midline of the body, circling the lips, and ending in the eyes.

The Governor Vessel meridian begins in the pelvic cavity where one branch goes up into the kidney, while the main line runs up the middle of the spinal column, enters the brain, flows up over the head, runs down the forehead and nose, and ends in the upper gums. Together the Conception and Governor Vessel meridians regulate the Yin (Conception Vessel) and Yang (Governor Vessel) of the whole body. When they are in harmony, powerful latent energies within the body are released, which rise along the central channel (Chong Mai) to the brain, nourishing the spirit and accelerating one's spiritual evolution.

Lung/Heart/Intestine Short Session

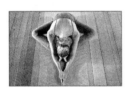 Butterfly Pose

 Quarter-Dog Pose

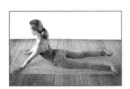 Seal Pose

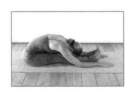 Full Forward Bend

 Child's Pose

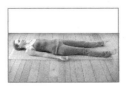 Corpse Pose (Savasana)

Butterfly Pose

This pose stimulates the Lung, Heart, and Small and Large Intestine meridians as we place pressure on the torso and abdomen folding forward (Fig.14.1). See page 38 for a full description of how to perform this pose.

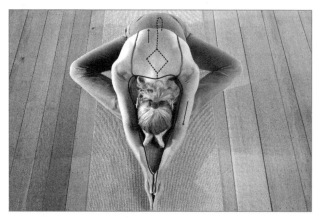

14.1. Butterfly Pose—Lung meridian shown

Seal Pose

This pose stimulates the Lung and Heart meridians as we lengthen the chest away from the abdomen and open the front of the body (Fig.14.2). See page 42 for a full description of how to perform this pose. You can also stimulate the pressure points in the fingers and affect each meridian in the upper body: the thumb is the Lung meridian, the first finger is the Large Intestine meridian, the middle finger is the Pericardium meridian, the ring finger is the Triple Heater meridian, and the small finger houses both the Heart and Small Intestine meridian points.

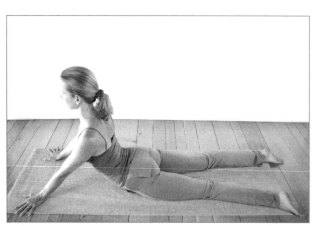

14.2. Seal Pose

Child's Pose

Do Child's Pose (Fig. 14.3) as described on page 42.

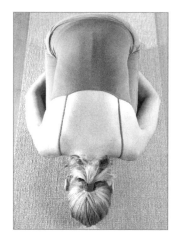

14.3. Child's Pose

Quarter-Dog Pose

This pose stimulates the Lung and Heart meridians as gentle pressure is placed across the shoulder joint and upper arms. Press into the fingers while doing this pose to stimulate the various points in each, as suggested in Seal Pose (Fig.14.4).

From Child's Pose, come forward onto all fours. Place your left forearm perpendicular to the upper arm and extend your right arm out, resting your elbow on the floor. Keep your hips back above your knees, which should be hip-width apart. Rest your head on the floor in front of your elbow or directly on the forearm. Allow your back to arch and your belly and underarms to drape toward the floor. If you have sensitivity in

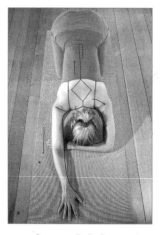

14.4. Quarter-Dog Pose—Lung meridian shown

your shoulders, place a cushion under your head to keep them higher (Fig. 14.5).

Stay in this pose for 3 to 5 minutes. To come out, inhale as you come back up to all fours. You can take a few breaths, rounding your spine, before changing sides. Rest in Child's Pose when you have completed both sides.

Full Forward Bend

This pose stimulates the Lung, Heart, and Intestine meridians as they flow through the torso and the abdominal region (which is under pressure) (Fig.14.6). See page 46 for a full description.

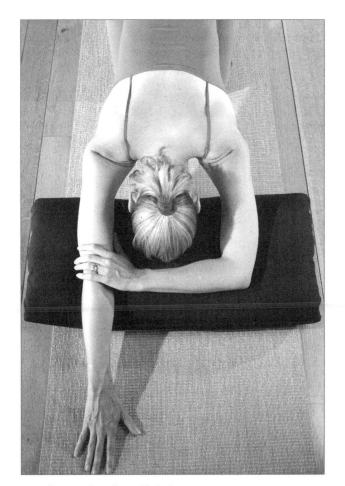

14.5. Quarter-Dog Pose, Variation

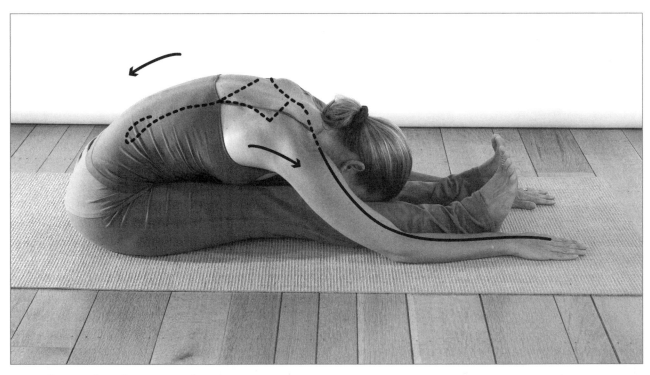

14.6. Full Forward Bend—Lung meridian shown

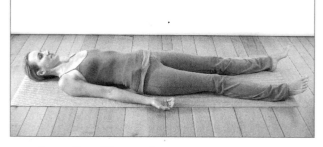

14.7. Corpse Pose (Savasana)

Corpse Pose (Savasana)

Do Corpse Pose (Savasana; Fig. 14.7) as described on page 47.

Lung/Heart/Intestine Long Session

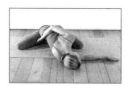 Wide-Knee Child's Pose with Twist (both sides)

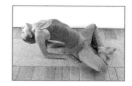 Full Forward Bend

 Sphinx Pose

 Snail Pose

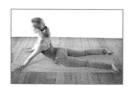 Seal Pose

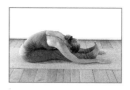 Fish Pose

 Child's Pose

 Lying Spinal Twist Pose (both sides)

 Quarter-Dog Pose

 Knees-into-the-Chest Pose

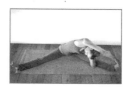 Lateral Dragonfly Pose

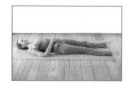 Corpse Pose (Savasana)

Wide-Knee Child's Pose with Twist

This pose stimulates the Lung, Heart, and Intestine meridians, as we twist to the side squeezing the abdominal region while opening the chest area (Fig.14.8). See page 76 for a full description of how to perform this pose.

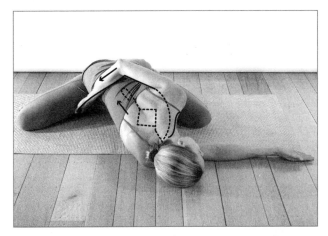

14.8. Wide-Knee Child's Pose with Twist—Lung meridian shown

Sphinx Pose

This pose, as well as Seal, stimulates the Lung, Heart, and Intestine meridians as they flow through the chest area, which is being lifted and widened, as well as in the abdominal region, which is being pulled into extension (Fig.14.9). See page 41 for a full description of how to perform this pose.

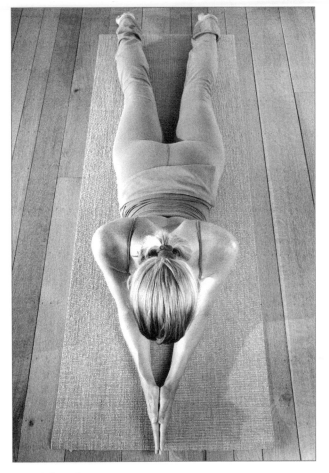

14.9. Sphinx Pose

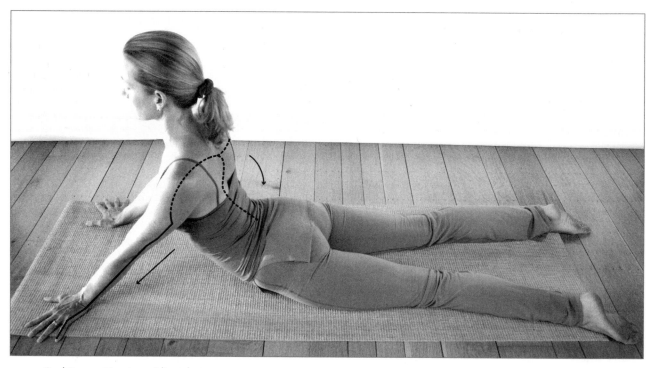

14.10. Seal Pose—Heart meridian shown

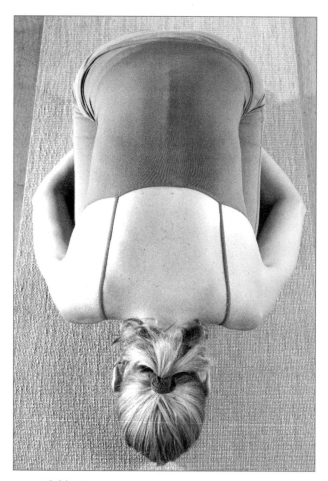

14.11. Child's Pose

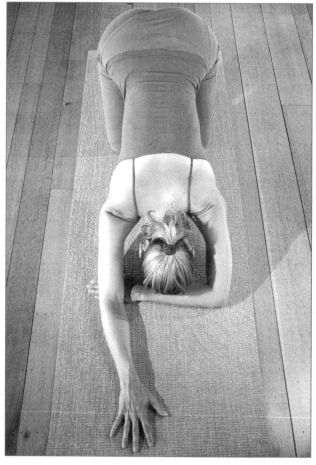

14.12. Quarter-Dog Pose

Seal Pose

Do Seal Pose (Fig. 14.10) as described on page 43.

Child's Pose

Enjoy Child's Pose (Fig. 14.11) as described on page 42.

Quarter-Dog Pose

Do Quarter-Dog Pose (Fig. 14.12) on both sides as described on page 92.

Lateral Dragonfly Pose

This pose stimulates the Lung, Heart, and Intestine meridians as you pull the tissues in the chest and abdomen over to one side, creating extended pressure on one side and elongation of the tissues on the opposite side, as well as pulling on the tissues along the shoulder and upper arm (Fig.14.13).

Sit straight with your legs in a wide straddle. Shift forward on your sitting bones and lean to the left, placing your left elbow on the floor along the inside of your leg, or on a cushion (Fig.14.14), and allowing your head to rest in your left hand. Your right hand can stay at your side, or you can rest your right arm across your head (or reach for your left foot with your right hand). Hold this pose for 3 to 5 minutes, then release your left elbow and rotate your torso so you are resting face-down over your left leg with your arms extended and relaxed on either side of the leg (Fig. 14.15).

Stay in this pose for 3 to 5 minutes. To come out, inhale and raise up. Bring your body back to center for a few breaths before repeating on the other side.

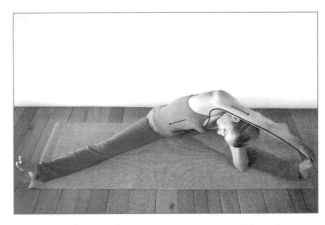

14.13. Lateral Dragonfly Pose, Part 1—Heart meridian shown

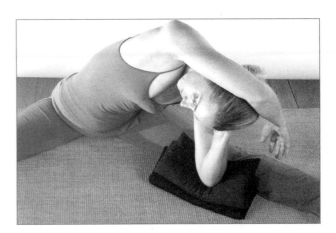

14.14. Lateral Dragonfly Pose, Variation

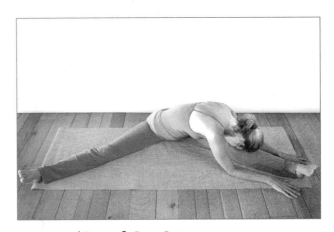

14.15. Lateral Dragonfly Pose, Part 2

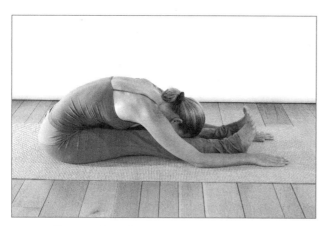

14.16. Full Forward Bend

Full Forward Bend

Do Full Forward Bend (Fig. 14.16) as described on page 46.

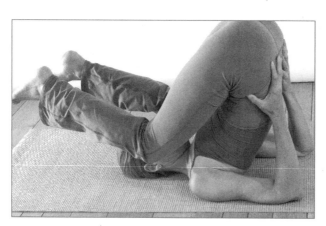

14.17. Snail Pose—Lung meridian shown

Snail Pose

This pose stimulates the Lung, Heart, and Intestine meridians as you compress the tissues in the chest and abdomen while elongating the tissues across the back (Fig. 14.17).

Lie on your back with your hands beside you. Inhale and bend your knees, bringing them over your head toward the floor. Keep your weight in your upper back rather than near your neck. If your feet drop down to the floor, lower your knees to the floor on either side of your head, grasping one wrist with the opposite hand on top of your calves. Allow your elbows to rest out to the side. Place your hands under your lower back if your feet do not rest on the floor (Fig. 14.18). Eliminate this pose from your sequence if you are in the first few days of your menstrual cycle, if you have infections in the head (such as sinus, eye, ear, or tooth infections), or if you have any neck sensitivity.

Stay in this pose for 3 to 5 minutes.

To come out, place your hands on the floor, and exhale as you roll your back to the floor, using your abdominals to slow you down and avoiding pressure on your neck. Bend your knees and place your feet on the floor while lying flat, moving your head slowly side to side. Stay here for a few breaths.

14.18. Snail Pose, Variation

Fish Pose

This pose stimulates the Lung, Heart, and Intestine meridians as you extend the tissues in the chest and abdomen while widening and opening the front of the body (Fig.14.19).

With your feet together as in Butterfly Pose, bring your elbows back under your shoulders to rest on the floor. Lift your chest while arching your back. Allow your head to drop back and rest on the trapezius muscles, or simply drop your head forward toward your chest. Keep your hands beside your hips.

Stay in this pose 2 to 3 minutes. To come out, move your elbows forward, then bring your chin to your chest and lie down. Extend your legs straight out.

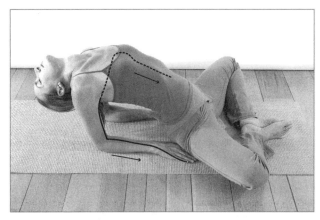

14.19. Fish Pose—Heart meridian shown

Lying Spinal Twist Pose

This pose stimulates the Lung, Heart, and Intestine meridians as you pressurize the back of the shoulder with the arm lifted above the body, widen along the chest, and squeeze the tissues in the abdomen (Fig.14.20). Follow the instructions on page 51, twisting to both sides. Stay 3 to 5 minutes on each side.

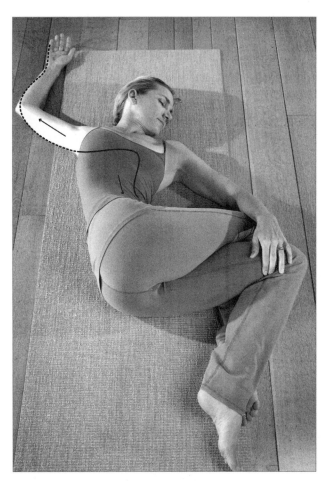

14.20. Lying Spinal Twist Pose—Heart meridian shown

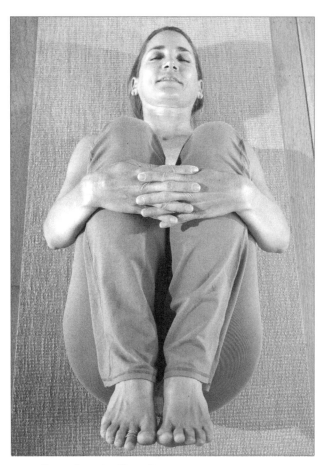
14.21. Knees-into-the-Chest Pose

Knees-into-the-Chest Pose

Lie on your back, bring both knees into your chest, and interlace your fingers around your shins (Fig. 14.21). Keep your sacrum, shoulders, and chin down.

Corpse Pose (Savasana)

Lie on your back with your arms and legs resting a few feet from center; turn your palms up. If your lower back has felt tight lately, place a blanket or bolster under the knees. You can also place a thin blanket under the head for added neck support and rest your hands on your abdomen if it's more comfortable than hands face up on the floor (Fig. 14.22). Rest in this pose 5 to 10 minutes.

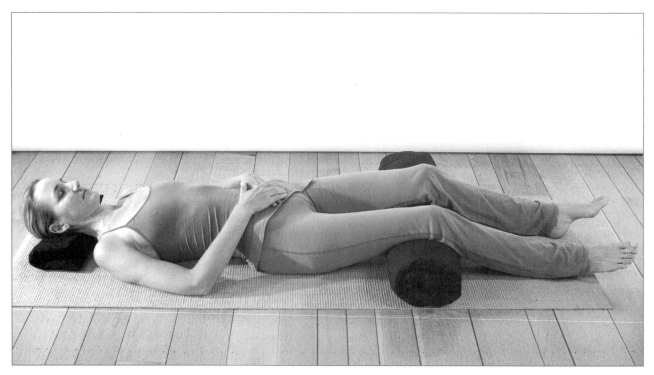
14.22. Corpse Pose (Savasana)

15

The Anatomy of the Mind in Yin Yoga

WE CAN NOW TURN OUR ATTENTION toward the anatomy of the mind in the Yin poses. We can begin each pose aligning our attention with the breath, then for the last few moments, relax into a noninterfering, meditative awareness. Beginning our practice with focused attention on the breath deepens our concentration, making it easier for thoughts to subside. When we rest in a nonstressful mental state, our energy body rebalances naturally. As our energy harmonizes, not only do our bodies open more easily, but our minds settle into an effortless contemplative repose, paving the way for meditative insight to occur.

Pranayama in Yin Yoga

Using our natural intelligence to focus on our breath and mobilize the distribution of prana throughout our body is called *pranayama,* which is an enhancement discipline that involves three aspects: inhalation (*puraka*); exhalation (*rechaka*); and the gap between, or suspension of breath (*kumbhaka*). By varying our respiration and holding our breath, we enhance the quality and motility of prana within. When practiced skillfully, intentional breathing has physical, energetic, and mental benefits. Physically, it helps oxygenate the blood and strengthens our digestive, eliminative, circulatory, and respiratory systems. Energetically, a pranayama practice helps balance, concentrate, and harmonize the flow of prana within us. When our energy is imbalanced, our prana is dissipated and weak, often resulting in unpredictable and dissonant emotions that leak out in uncontrolled, chaotic ways. A yogi, on the other hand, is described as someone whose prana is contained within the center of her body. Her emotional life is rich and her mind clear.

In pranayama, we attempt to reduce the amount of prana that leaks out and enliven the quality of energy existing within us. This is not possible without concentration. Our mind is closely linked to the quality of our prana, and our breath influences our pranic body. When we concentrate on using our breath to balance the subtle (or energy) body, there is a unifying effect on our overall state of being.

Through aligning our minds with our breath, we can experience relaxed alertness in the energy body and mind, a state that has extremely therapeutic effects on the body. The key ingredient is attention. As we watch the breath, we begin to tune in to our capacity for focus and concentration, qualities that arouse meditative awareness. Pranayama is therefore a wonderful practice to sequence before meditation, because it tethers the mind and prana within our body, amplifying our awareness in the present moment.

The breath can be thought of as the catalyst for inner circulation. When we engage in full use of our diaphragm in an unhurried and conscious way, we assist in enhancing the distribution of prana throughout our bodies. This style of breathing is called Ujjayi ("victorious") breath and has a number of benefits. As we slow down the rhythm of each breath, it has a soothing effect on our nervous system. This in turn releases the tensions in our body, helping us to feel more relaxed. As we let go, we tune in to the sound of our breathing, helping to diminish the distractions of the mind and leading to more inner quietude. Focusing on the breath in this way helps increase our ability to concentrate in an effortless manner, preparing the body and mind for deeper integration. Please turn to page 107 to learn more about this method.

Now that you understand Ujjayi breathing, you can refine three aspects to it. Allow your attention to focus on the length, depth, and direction of each breath. Begin to slow the length of your breath to about 5 seconds for an inhalation, staying aware of the stillness of breath that ensues at the end of the inhalation, then make the exhalation the same length (about 5 seconds). Be aware of the rest space that occurs as your lungs empty completely.

There are four beats to which you need to stay attentive. The first is the movement of the inhalation; the second is the rest space after you have filled up with air. The third beat is the movement of the exhalation, and the fourth is the quietude that occurs after all the air has escaped and before the next breath is born. As you listen to the breath in this way, learn to stay attentive to both that which is obvious (the movement of breath) and that which is subtle (the formless space between breaths), breeding insight into the constant interplay between movement and stillness.

Allow this rhythm to continue without straining as you listen to the smoothness of the breath,

softening any areas where you notice that it sounds labored, pushed, or staccato. The second feature to be aware of about the breath is its depth. The sound of the breath will help you detect how deep it is. When you breathe superficially, force the breath, or are unconscious of your breath, it will sound like an out-of-tune wind instrument whose notes stumble along disharmoniously. We are becoming artists of the breath, listening with the same precision that musicians do when tuning up for a concert. As you even out the sound from the beginning, into the middle, and all the way to the end of each breath, you will naturally and effortlessly deepen it. It will sound more like a distant river, steady and clear.

Having aligned the length and depth of breath, we can now focus on the third feature—the direction. As we inhale, the conventional pattern of our in-breath is to expand our lungs and move our energy up and out. Yogis call this upward pattern or wind the prana vayu. As we exhale, the conventional pattern of our out-breath is to contract the respiratory muscles and move our energy down and out. This downward pattern or wind is called the apana vayu. A yoga practitioner has the potential to enliven these two inner circulations by preventing them from leaving the body and directing them instead to move toward each other and toward the center of the body. This is accomplished by using the mind and imagination to move the upward wind down as we inhale, while raising the downward wind up when we exhale.

The technique is quite simple. As you inhale for a slow 5-minute interval, feel the breath coming in and move your awareness down along the center of your body to your pelvic floor. Draw your perineum (between the anus and the genitals) slightly in, as if magnetizing the inhalation on its way down. Now that you are at the end of the inhalation, your attention should be down at the bottom of your spine, feeling a subtle suctioning at the base, which is called the mula. In this way, the perineum acts as a chi bridge and redirects the downward dissipation of energy back into the center of the body, refining the quality of both the prana and apana winds by joining them, causing more enhanced chi throughout the center of the body. This drawing-in action at the pelvic floor is traditionally called Root Lock

(Mula bandha; see page 164). As the exhalation begins, springboard off your perineum like bouncing off a trampoline, and propel the energy back up toward your heart center, ending the exhalation where you began, in your chest.

This movement down on the inhalation and up on the exhalation encourages a better absorption of chi into the center of the body, thereby enhancing our vitality while helping to concentrate our minds. Continue this breath awareness discipline on the length, depth, and direction of breath for the first two to three minutes of each pose.

Breath Retentions and Chakra Visualizations

The meridian channels within the body get their vitality from the vortex centers along the central channel called chakras. These centers are considered cauldrons of energy by the Taoists, places where psychic forces and bodily functions merge. The chakras collect, transform, and distribute energy throughout the system. They are the junction between the form body and the energetic, formless dimensions. They are the lungs of the energy body, and each vibrating disk has specific functions that affect our overall well-being in various ways.

Yogis suggest that our basic physical and mental health is dependant on the natural functionality of each chakra. Although their fundamental capacity depends on our constitution, they can be activated and enlivened by mental concentration. As they are the source or wellspring of the energy body, when they lack full vibrancy and are impaired, our physical and mental health will suffer.

When we are already sick, revitalizing the chakra that is responsible for that function will have a direct effect on our body's capacity to rebalance. There are many ancient and often secret practices that affect the chakras. These disciplines are called awakening the chakras and should only be attempted under the guidance of a qualified master. Here we will focus on simple concentration and visualization techniques that are safe to do while in Yin poses to improve specific basic functions of the chakras and the meridians they nourish.

Chakras are generators of prana, intersection sites where heightened pranic activity takes place;

the prana is then channeled via the meridians to all the regions of the body. Amplifying chakra activity is accomplished through the use of mental concentration and visualization. It has already been mentioned that refined prana will gather at places in the body on which we focus without distraction. This process is enhanced if we concentrate on particular areas after we have completed the inhalation or exhalation process—in other words, during the suspension of breath. If we are interested in affecting one of the chakras below the ribs, it is best to concentrate on this area during forward bends as the area is being pressured by the pose, as well as at the end of an exhalation, concentrating the effect in the lower abdominal region where these chakras dwell. The practice of holding the breath after exhalation is called *langhana,* which refers to a capacity to reduce, and has a beneficial effect on the organs in the abdominal region as well as the lower chakras. If you have issues with your digestive, eliminative, or reproductive organs, or with the kidney, spleen, or liver chi, you should practice this method during the Yin yoga sequences for those three meridians.

If we are interested in affecting one of the chakras above the navel, it is best to focus on them during backbends, after a full inhalation, when the chi is more concentrated in the chest and upper regions. This practice is called *brmhana,* which refers to the capacity to expand. This practice has an energizing and warming effect on the body and can be helpful for issues related to the circulatory or respiratory systems, as well as the lungs, heart, or intestines. *Brmhana* can be practiced in the yin yoga sequences for these meridians as well.

It is important to remember that if after holding the breath, you notice that the next breath you take is greatly reduced or labored, then stop. Respiration and heart rate are interdependent, and if your breathing is poor, your pulse will go up, which can be risky. We should always feel at ease when practicing pranayama, able to calmly observe the quality of each breath.

Chakra Visualizations

Each energy vortex has particular functions on both the physical and the psychological levels. The

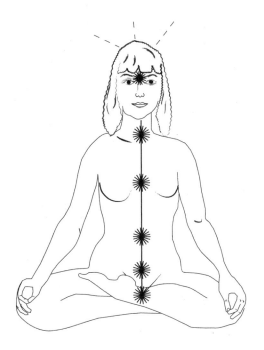

following is a brief explanation of each chakra and how to focus attention on each of them.

Muladhara

Mula means "root," and *dhara* means "base." The muladhara is located above the anus, near the perineum or cervix. It relates to our dormant inner power,* our sense of security, our material drive, and elimination. It is also related to the Kidney, Urinary Bladder, and Small Intestine meridians.

Svadishthana

Svadishthana literally means "one's own abode." This chakra is located above and behind the genitals and sacral region. This area relates to our sensual and sexual drives; our unconscious material, as well as the collective unconscious. It governs all reproductive issues; intuition; and the Kidney, Urinary Bladder, and Small Intestine meridians and their functions.

Manipura

Manipura means "filled with jewels." It is located behind the navel, corresponding to the solar plexus. This area houses the seat of our willpower, creative energy, imagination, and digestion. It rules the digestive meridians, including those of the stomach, spleen, liver, and gallbladder.

Anahata

Anahata means "unbroken." This chakra is located to the right of the physical heart. It relates to our drive for love and compassion, our circulatory system, and our sense of touch. It rules the Heart and Pericardium meridians.

Vishuddhi

Vishuddhi means "to purify." This chakra is located at the throat and it relates to our spiritual drive, our ability to communicate, and our respiratory system. It rules the Lung meridian.

Ajna

Ajna means " to know." It is located in the brain core, midway between the eyebrows, and is often called the third eye. It relates to our intelligence, insight, and clarity; our autonomic nervous system, and our hormonal system. It governs the Governor Vessel and Urinary Bladder meridians.

Sahasrara

Sahasrara means "thousand-petaled lotus." It is located at the crown of the head, and it governs our cerebral cortex, our entire nervous system, and the organs and tissues of our entire body. It also relates to a highly refined quality of mind resting in a non-dual consciousness known as One Taste. It is not connected with any specific meridian, but to all of them.

Method for Lower Chakra Enhancement

While in any seated forward bend, such as Butterfly Pose or Shoelace Pose, bring your attention to guiding each inhalation down your body toward your perineum, while bringing the exhalation back up to your chest. Decide whether you need to focus more on issues related to elimination and feeling grounded (focus on the first chakra at your perineum); reproductive issues and/or intuition

---

*This creative force is referred to as a sleeping serpent at the base of our spine called the Kundalini. When the Kundalini begins to awaken, this force is referred to as Shakti, the feminine source energy of all natural, universal evolutionary processes. The purpose of practices that attempt to "awaken" the chakras is to release this potent but dormant energy within to transform the body and mind into more and more refined functions and levels of consciousness. See *Awakening the Chakras and Emancipation* by Dr. Hiroshi Motoyama for further exploration on this subject.

(focus on the second chakra in your lower belly); or digestive and/or energetic and creative concerns (focus on the third chakra behind your navel).

On an exhalation, after you have emptied out the breath completely, bring your attention to one of these three sites and abide there for 2 or 3 seconds. Then allow your inhalation to begin again with your attention focused at your chest and moving down toward your pelvic floor. Exhale and again ride up the center of the body as you empty of air. After the end of the exhalation, pause again for a few seconds in the same chakra area. Continue this way for 2 to 3 minutes as you hold the pose. If you are staying for a five-minute interval, rest your attention in a relaxed awareness for the remaining few minutes (see chapters 16 and 20 for more on mindfulness in Yin yoga).

As you begin the next pose, if it is also a forward bend (or the other side of an asymmetrical pose), repeat the same technique, allowing for the first few minutes to be a focused pranayama and chakra visualization practice, and the last few minutes to be practiced with a restful but alert attention throughout your whole body. If you have a few areas you would like to address in one session, you can alternate which chakra you focus on in each pose.

Method for Upper Chakra Enhancement

While in Saddle Pose, Sphinx Pose, or Seal Pose, bring your attention to guiding the inhalation down your body toward your perineum and to bringing the exhalation back up to your chest (you can also practice this method in Snail Pose or Fish Pose). Decide whether you need to focus more on issues related to the circulatory system and feelings of wounded love, depression, lack of warmth, or hatred (focus on the fourth chakra in your heart); the respiratory system, and feelings of uncertainty in your spiritual life, or communication issues (focus on the fifth chakra at your throat); or hormonal issues, bladder dysfunctions, or a lack of alertness, clarity, or insight (focus on the sixth chakra between your eyes).

On an inhalation, travel from your chest to your pelvic floor as you have been doing. After you have filled up with breath completely, bring your attention to one of these three sites and remain there for 2 or 3 seconds before allowing the exhalation. Then

bring your attention back to your perineum area, and exhale from there up to your chest again. At the end of the next inhalation, pause again for a few seconds in the same chakra area. Continue this way for 2 to 3 minutes as you hold the pose. If you are staying in it for a 5-minute interval, rest your attention in a relaxed awareness for the remaining few minutes.

Mindfulness in Yin Yoga

We can now proceed from this kind of focusing (which is useful to concentrate prana into various parts of the body and help these areas rebalance) to a more relaxed kind of concentration. Prana becomes quite disturbed and unbalanced if we compulsively and unceasingly guide its direction or constantly react to the play of emotional and mental states. With a relaxed concentration, a mental equilibrium is achieved that has an immediate harmonizing effect on the energy and emotional body. With constant intervention we fail to recognize the unstained nature of mind, where nothing need be added or corrected.

Mindfulness is not an enhancement discipline per se. It is an attitude we adopt in which we let go of all motivations to manipulate the moment and develop the capacity to observe without any willful interference. With practice, this refined quality of attention causes three distinct changes in us. The first is that our fragmented, distracted habits of mind begin to diminish. This helps us understand ourselves and others with greater honesty and clarity. The second effect is that our negative and aggressive afflictions are diffused, changing our behavior patterns. This occurs not by suppressing them, but by viewing them with an inquisitive attitude of interest and inclusion. Third, our essential or authentic nature, disentangled from reactive patterns of the personality, becomes revealed and accessible. As we strip away the identifications and reactions to which we usually adhere, what shines through is our inherent open dimension of being.

After a few minutes of focused concentration on the breath (as described in the preceding sections), open into a relaxed concentration in which you allow your attention to remain aware of the particular sensations in your body (as well as feelings and thoughts in your mind, sounds and temperature in the room, and so on), without interfering with anything that is noticed. Don't try to minimize or embellish any aspect. Instead, remain fairly still in your pose, engendering an increased willingness to experience this moment without any psychological resistance. If you begin struggling with the sensations, allow yourself to directly observe each aspect of tension—physical as well as mental—with an interest in suspending the judgment that you should be feeling something else (unless, of course, you perceive the sensations as sharp, electrical, or nerve tingling, in which case, back out of the pose).

Let your attention go into your hips or lower back, wherever the sensation is strongest, and observe it fully. Does it have a shape, a temperature, and a texture? As you are both looking at and feeling what is happening, notice if the sensation is vibrating in any way, changing from breath to breath or moment to moment. Can you observe the subtlety of change in the seemingly solid blockage without imposing or manipulating—just being there with it? This is a surrendering practice. Rest assured that as the minutes unfold, your ability to be nonresistant to physical limitations will become more challenging. But as it becomes more intense, and you stay with the practice, a courageous maturity can unfold through your consistent willingness to stay present and nonreactive in the face of challenging sensations and/or emotions.

The important attitude here is willingness rather than willfulness. We are not hardening inside waiting for the time to end so we can come out of the pose and feel okay again. We are heightening our capacity to feel alert and at ease, despite challenging physical and psychological discomforts. If the sensations are too much and you are feeling overwhelmed by them, then it is skillful to back out of the pose a bit to diminish the intensity so you can continue your mind training.

This cultivation of bare attention is the foundation of a mindfulness practice. As we begin to soften in the face of challenging (but not overly threatening) physical limitations, we may discover a portal into an unlimited supply of psychological openness. This attitude has a direct harmonizing quality on our body. It also becomes the doorway into freeing the mind of its assumed limitations, its strategies of evasion, or the habit of controlling or struggling with our experience. We may eventu-

ally learn that despite the strong sensations in our hip and/or groin while in Butterfly Pose, the mind can be at rest—clear and attentive.

At times you may feel the blockage in your outer hip as anger (related to gallbladder disharmonies), or fear (the emotion related to kidneys) may arise as you linger in the backbends. Staying connected to what is arising inside you without acting out from these feelings allows them space to breathe, to move, to be experienced as less solid and therefore less threatening. They are no longer stuffed back down into unawareness, becoming fertile ground for future reactivity given the proper stimulus. Instead, they become beacons of growth, nudging us into widening our capacity to include difficulty on the path of full awareness, liberating our patterns of habitual armor or defense, moment by moment.

We are learning to track the sensations moving through us, giving particular attention to the ones to which we feel resistant. If we notice hostility within, our focus shifts from the physical sensation to observing our feelings of aversion to these sensations or of craving others. Instead of ignoring this dimension of our experience, craving or aversion becomes the object of our attention. Our emotional afflictions can become avenues to deepening wisdom when they are worked with in a skillful way.

As we observe difficult feelings moving through us, we bathe them in nonabandoning attention, softening our identification with the struggle. As these feelings are not solid "things," the energy they feed on for substantiality is our hardened mind states. As we relax the struggle with them, they become empty and inevitably dissipate.

We may still have the same amount of physical pain and discomfort, but we are no longer suffering the pain in the same way. As we let go of the suffering, we begin to foster a continued intimacy with our moments, regardless of what shows up in them (whether painful, neutral, or pleasant), diminishing our ingrained habits to cling to, fight, or disconnect from our experience. The Yin practice, with its inherently challenging physical component and often retaliatory and uncomfortable feelings, is an optimal place to develop these qualities of mindfulness and meditative awareness. Please see chapters 19 and 20 to help expand your capacity to strengthen meditative awareness in your Yin practice.

16

Yang Yoga (Dynamic Flow)

J UST AS YIN YOGA has particular gifts that arise when we practice sincerely, Yang yoga—or an active practice—will develop qualities that a more receptive, quieter practice cannot. All areas of the body need to be used in order to maintain their functionality, so we must mobilize the active aspect of the energy body (residing in the more superficial tissues) regularly to refresh the body's alert vibrancy and maintain its health. This will not only keep our bodies functional and comfortable throughout our lives, but it will also teach us how to directly inhabit all the subtleties of this form body in an engaging way. However, because this practice resembles sports, dance, and gymnastics, it is important to carry over mindful attitudes from the Yin style. This will help us respect our limitations, avoiding the competition and comparison so common in other physical disciplines.

Since there are so many features to contend with when movement is involved, it is easier to develop unskillful ways of being during this practice period. We need to be on high alert for the potential to slip into aggressive attitudes, performance anxiety, or competitive comparisons to others and our own abilities in the past. For this reason, I often find starting with the Yin style of practice very helpful in setting an inner tone of compassionate attention.

There are seven key concepts with which we need to become familiar before we begin moving into active yoga poses, or asanas. These ideas are actually inner actions that set up an inner alignment, creating the foundation for outer or postural alignment. The first four are physical/energetic and the last three are psychological:

> Ujjayi breathing
> Breathing into our edge
> Lines of energy
> Tensegrity
> Respecting our limitations
> Equanimity of interest
> Willingness to feel

Ujjayi Breathing

This is a deep, diaphragmatic breath that is often translated as "the victorious stretching of the inner breath." Ujjayi breathing has a number of benefits that are helpful to inspire us to practice it when we are in our yoga sessions. This slow and deep style of breathing strengthens our lungs and diaphragm, while allowing a deeper intake of oxygen and full expulsion of carbon dioxide, enriching the blood. Ujjayi breathing also slows down the passage of air, having a calming effect on our nervous system. As this happens, our body relaxes and the mind quiets, allowing us to melt into the yoga postures much more graciously. This type of breathing also creates a steady, sonorous sound that becomes a barometer for how we are working with ourselves and acts as an anchor to keep the mind focused in the present.

To learn Ujjayi breathing, sit in a comfortable position with your spine elongated and your sitting bones resting evenly on a cushion. Close your eyes and become aware of your breath. Notice if your belly raises or contracts on the inhalations. Notice what happens on the exhalations. Now consciously draw your belly in toward your spine on your next exhalation, and allow it to relax on the inhalation. This may be different than what you have been doing, so place one hand on your belly to remind yourself to pull it back gently as you breathe out. This is the first piece to connect with in Ujjayi breathing.

The second aspect involves slowing down the passage through which the air travels in order to take longer breaths. The narrower the tunnel, the longer you will take to fill up completely with air. A longer breath is what triggers the relaxation response in the nervous system, so it is preferable to inhale slowly rather than swiftly right now. To slow this passage of air, we close off part of our throat (the glottis, or space between the vocal chords) and breathe predominantly through the back of the throat. This is natural and something you do every time you whisper.

Although this breathing style is done through the nostrils, it is helpful to learn it first through the mouth, focusing on the exhalation. To create this slower rhythm, first take an inhalation and as you begin the exhalation, open your mouth and say, "Whisper," extending the "r" sound. Inhale again and on the next exhalation, simply repeat the "r" sound through the back of your throat, without the use of your vocal chords. After an-

other inhalation, begin the exhalation with your mouth open, making the "r" sound, and halfway through, close your mouth and breathe through your nose while continuing to make the sound in the back of your throat. It will sound like waves starting under the ocean or wind moving through trees. You do not need to project it very loudly. It will be softly audible to you but probably not very perceptible to someone right next to you. Remember, this style of breathing can greatly help you regulate how to work with yourself nonaggressively, yet it may become slightly louder when you are in an active practice.

Continue to keep your mouth closed now and see if you can make the same sound on the inhalation as well, pulling the air in slowly through the back of your throat. If you can only do it on the exhalation, don't worry. It is easier for most people on the exhalation first. After a few days or weeks of practice, you will undoubtedly be able to breathe in the same way on the inhalation also. If you lose the rhythm or start to pant, stop and take a few ordinary breaths. Begin the process again with the open-mouth exhalation and the soft sound as you breathe out each time. It should become less arduous and more effortless with practice. If you continue to feel frustrated trying to figure this out, seek out a yoga teacher and go through the process together.

Once you feel comfortable with it, breathe only through your nose and see if you can allow the breath to travel in and out even more slowly. Try to breathe in for 4 to 6 seconds and make the exhalation the same length. Maintaining this way of breathing as you move through yoga postures will help prevent any overaggression or unconscious striving, precursors to most injuries. Allow your breath to be the most important element of your practice now, backing off or coming out of a pose to rest when you notice your breath has sped up or sounds jagged or forced.

Breathing into Our Edge

The next vital component is moving the breath into various parts of the body, often called "breathing into an edge." This inner action involves focusing our breath through our imagination into various places in our body. Remember, where our attention goes, prana flows. We are interested in waking up all the inner tissues, using our breath awareness to rebalance and enliven each natural range of motion. As our primary mental focus is placed on the breath and into various body parts, we learn to discern how far to deepen into each area and when to yield and surrender to the resistance felt. Moving into a pose from breath awareness allows us to go in slowly, with respect and care, sensitive to our body's feedback signals moment to moment. This responsiveness develops the necessary discernment between risky pain (to be avoided) and unavoidable discomfort (constrictive and weak sensations we have to be willing to feel to bring these areas to life).

Without breath awareness, we are much more likely either to give up at the first hint of intense sensations (causing us to miss the gift of discovering and living in uncharted territory) or to strain. When we are overly hesitant and afraid about feeling uncomfortable as we enter a pose and experience resistance in our bodies, we are forgetting that in order to wake up the various places of immobility inside, we have to reenter these areas repeatedly, reinhabiting them over and over again. This means we have to be willing to go through the discomfort in them before we experience the joy of aliveness in them.

Without a clear focus on the breath leading us slowly into our bodies to an appropriate edge, we may plunge in with overambitious enthusiasm, unwittingly bypassing an appropriate limitation and thrashing forward with aggressive fixation. With the breath as our primary guide, we gradually move into ever-deepening realms of sensitivity and possibility, learning to avoid the extremes of under- or overuse in any area.

To learn breathing into your edge, stay in the sitting position you used for Ujjayi breathing and allow a slow, conscious breath to continue. Take a breath in, and on the exhalation, walk your hands onto the floor in front of you, keeping your sitting bones grounded but allowing your arms and spine to extend forward as far as they can without strain. When you can't go any farther because of your knees, hips, or lower back, pause and take

a few Ujjayi breaths. Envision the breath specifically entering the areas where you feel strong sensations. This is your first edge. You may notice after a short while that the initial tension has subsided and you can draw your hands out a little bit farther now—so do. This is your second edge. Again, after a few breaths, you may feel the organic impulse to drop deeper in, or you may sense a blockage somewhere else, so you back off from this edge.

In this way, breath to breath, we sense where our natural limitations are and send the breath into the places we feel most intensely. Often, as we come into these poses, our edges will drop more and more, bit by bit. At other times, as we rest a while to acclimatize to a shape, we will feel other areas talking back to us, and our edge will need to back off so these pockets can release before they build up too much pressure within them.

Lines of Energy

Lines of energy are like shooting rays of light or electricity through the internal pathways, the meridians. Along with breathing into our edge by placing the breath in a specific area, engaging lines of energy requires that we place our attention on the lines our body is forming in each posture and extend the feeling of vibrancy out beyond our physical form. We can begin to imagine that as we breathe in vital chi and circulate it through our system, we can also send out vibrant energetic currents through the subtle body highways. This allows us to experience the yoga shapes from the inside out. When we are conscious of receiving and sending rivers of energy coordinated with the breathing process, we experience our body as much lighter, more fluid, and more able to endure difficult positions without the hindrance of overt heaviness.

You can think of these rays as originating in your belly when sending the lines down and out through the legs, and as stemming from your heart center when directing them through your shoulders and out your arms and fingers. To put this into practice, simply sit upright in a comfortable, cross-legged position. Bring your right arm out at shoulder height with the palm facing down. Begin your Ujjayi breathing while focusing all your attention in the center of your chest. Imagine that a ball of energy in your heart center begins to flow out into your shoulder, creating an electrical highway through your arm. Keep breathing while imagining the energy pouring through your upper arm, your elbow, your forearm, and into your wrist. As you continue breathing, send this energy pulsation out your hand and through space as far as you can imagine. You have created one line of energy. Feel the current and aliveness you have brought to your arm via your attention through it.

Keeping your right arm in the air, raise your left arm and shift all of your focus into that highway of energy. Send a flow of attention from your chest through your left shoulder and elbow and out your hand. Notice how heavy your right arm feels in contrast to your left. While maintaining the left line of energy, reengage the flow through the right. Your right arm, although tired from being elevated so long, will no doubt feel lighter when your attention streams through it as compared to when it doesn't. You now have two lines of energy moving in opposite directions, or you could say one line of energy that is bidirectional. Most lines of energy have a force of attention streaming in one direction and simultaneously pulsing the other way as well. Bring your arms down and notice the sensations in your upper body. As you sit upright, you can imagine a line of energy moving up from your chest and out your spine, and another originating in your navel center that flows down and out into the floor. So in any position you find yourself, you can discover how many lines your body shape is creating and simply direct shooting rays of light into those pathways with your imagination. You can envision bringing in rays of light toward your energy centers on an inhalation and sending out energy lines on the exhalation from your chest or belly center—or both. Whenever you find yourself feeling dense and drained of vitality in a pose, instead of immediately coming out, check to see if you are practicing energetic guidance through the shape. Most likely you are not. Realign your attention with the energetic experience, and watch how

much stronger your endurance becomes, as well as your joy in experiencing the postures.

Tensegrity

Tensegrity is a term used in architecture that describes integral tension between components in a three-dimensional structure. Buckminster Fuller explained that compression and tension (push and pull) are not opposites, but coessential complements that are inseparable. Tensegrity describes how all structures maintain their integral shape when appropriate tensile and compressive factors complement each other.

Carlos Castaneda used the term to refer to a practice called magical passes (which involve slow, contemplative postures and movements). He used this term because, like yoga, the magical passes involve engaging and relaxing the muscles and joints to encourage greater body consciousness.

As we create a dynamic pose, tensegrity applies in numerous areas of our body as we continually pull one area closer together while drawing another area farther apart. As one area moves in, another area close by needs to move out. As one area lifts, the opposing area needs to descend. When something is extended forward, there is always an opposing force moving back. Learning how to integrate these polar actions smoothly is an ever-deepening art that requires exposure to skillful teachers, as well as a committed regular practice.

Respecting Our Limitations

As we begin to move into our bodies in an active way—tugging the tissues in one direction, pulling them in another—we immediately face our body's blockages and incapacities. As we meet these strengthening and lengthening limitations, the most important part of the experience is not whether or not we can perform a certain posture, but rather our attitude toward ourselves as we feel each pose. Yang asana requires us to develop sensitivity in action, patiently discovering the appropriate amount of energy to work with moment by moment. Practicing Yin yoga first gives us an opportunity to heighten our responsiveness to our internal feedback, acting on the signals we receive about how far to go into a pose rather than using force or willfulness. When these same sensibilities are translated into the Yang practice, we develop a natural curiosity and respect for our body that is essential not only for the chi to flow freely, but also for us to grow into an ongoing love affair with embodiment.

We are "practicing" living in our bodies in an honorable and dignified way, free of the constricting entrapment of competition or ambition (qualities that are appropriate in other contexts but create havoc when allowed to bleed into our yoga practice). We must develop this discerning attitude in order to progress to greater levels of self-care and sanity. With the breath as our primary anchor, we can learn to listen to variations in its tone in order to wake up to the mechanical reactions that arise when we feel physical limitations.

If we remember that we are literally looking for these blockages in each pose so as to delicately inhabit them again, then we will feel less threatened when they reveal themselves. They do not actually cause us to suffer; it is our attitude about them that determines whether or not we will graciously turn toward what needs attention or turn away. This willingness to feel our pains and bring fresh attention there is one of the most life-affirming capacities that a physical-based yoga practice can help us develop, causing us to translate this body-based consciousness into more and more moments throughout our day.

Equanimity of Interest

Equanimity is a word that describes a lack of partiality—in other words, evenness. In our yoga practice, it refers to a telescopic approach toward ourselves that is all-inclusive. Each shape we take is an opportunity to spread our attention globally throughout the form we are in. We may be feeling an enormous amount of weight on one leg as we lunge forward in Warrior I Pose, but our field of attention encompasses both an awareness of the places under stress (the front quadriceps), as well as the places without weight in them (the torso, arms, and hands). We are developing the capacity to track the sensations continuously from head to toe, sending the distribution of energy to where it is most needed, while continuing to feel the more subtle flows elsewhere.

This constant maintenance of our energy refines our mental acuity, enlivening our ability to stay interested and connected to the ever-changing sensations that each posture creates. We develop a capacity to widen our scope of bodily awareness beyond those sensations that merely bring us comfort and pleasure, releasing our compulsions to seek and expect only easy, pleasant sensations. In fact, instead of wishing it were easier, we look for the possibility of finding ease within challenging circumstances.

An equanimity of interest means we are just as turned on by the experience of restricted hamstrings in Downward-Facing Dog Pose (Adho Mukha Svanasana) as we are by the capacity to effortlessly maintain our balance in a one-legged Bridge Pose. As we wake up our bodies each day, we undoubtedly experience a wide array of feelings no matter how accomplished our practice is. The difference between a beginner and an adept is less about postural ability and much more about the breadth of interest in attending, regardless of what limitations are discovered.

Willingness to Feel

For any of the other concepts to be put into practice, we have to cultivate a willingness to feel if we are to discover what it means to live an embodied wholeness. Whether we feel lousy or exuberant, tight or agile, we need to reinvest daily in a commitment to let ourselves be assaulted or bemused without becoming oppressed by these feelings. We are training ourselves to stay connected to what is happening within us without retaliating or abandoning the scene.

As we drop down into our bodily experience, we have to be willing to feel all the places we have vacated or abused in the past in order to bring the life force back into them. This behavior is a loving and courageous act. Without a conscious commitment to enliven ourselves through a daily yoga practice (regardless of what has happened in the past or how incapable we feel), we are lulled back into our unconscious habits of emotional armoring, carelessness, and neglect. It is so easy to discard our best intentions when we are uncomfortable, feel lazy, or are just overly busy. The willingness to feel into our bodies daily reminds us afresh that we value living in an inclusive and conscious way. This kind of consistent care causes us to acknowledge and eventually abandon mechanical behavior that inevitably deadens us to deep feeling tones. We all have various degrees of emotional scarring and woundedness that our survival personality traits constantly try to manage. The precious gift of a skillful daily practice is that we learn that we can actually alter the course of any situation (regardless of our past), when we remain awake and aware in a nonreactive way.

17

Yang Sequences for Balancing with a Yin Practice

THERE ARE MANY WAYS to approach a Yang practice. I have found that the more interested I am in balancing Yin and Yang in my physical practice, the more my Yang practice needs to address developing a core strength and mobility in the muscles to complement all the ways I have pulled my skeleton apart during my Yin practice. Recognizing that unlike yin tissues, yang tissues love rhythmic movement, I often begin with simple, repetitive movements like Sun Salutations (Surya Namaskar) to increase the fluid content in the tissues and develop an alert focus on Ujjayi breathing.

What follows are four skillful sequences, one for beginners or people wanting a less vigorous practice, and three others that can be intensified depending on how many repetitions you do of each pose. The practice for beginners integrates Yin and Yang styles and will develop deeper body awareness and energetic integrity. I find it more helpful to put the Yang poses first for brand-new beginners because the movement practice settles the mind and nervous system enough to begin the more challenging training of holding Yin poses for a bit longer. The focus of this practice is to bring your awareness into the center or core of your body in an active way first. This allows the Yin poses at the end of the session (done on your back for hip elasticity and meridian health) to help you begin to develop a meditative attention.

Those with more skill and energy may appreciate the concise and well-balanced sequence of Sun Salutation (Surya Namaskar) that can be completed in fifteen minutes or extended to a longer session. This complete Yang practice complements long Yin sessions very well by promoting structural strength and stability in all the areas you open in the Yin style. The third sequence focuses on nourishing the Kidney organ-meridian pair by attracting chi to the lower torso and developing core strength. It is a good practice when you want to soothe the entire system, feel centered and invigorated in yourself, and keep the intensity level down. The last session warms the body and impacts the heart and small intestine organ-meridian pairs with an even distribution of energy in the lower and upper body with standing poses and inversions. Standing poses bring needed strength, length, and grounding to the lower body, while inversions are an irreplaceable way of enhancing blood flow to the brain; stimulating the lymphatic, digestive, and eliminative systems; and maintaining elasticity and tone in the veins and arteries. This session demands more vigor and skill, but when practiced in combination with Yin poses and meditation, it will keep your body and mind vibrant and enlivened.

When you practice these four Yang sequences regularly in concert with a Yin practice and meditation, you create a natural congruency between your upper and lower, inner and outer, yin and yang aspects of body and mind. You then truly align yourself with the possibility for embodied wholeness.

Yang/Yin Session for Beginners

Yang Poses

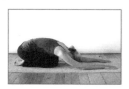 Child's Pose (Adho Mukha Virasana)

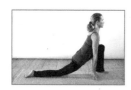 Ruddy Goose Pose (Chakravakasana)

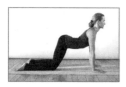 Lunge Pose with Hands Down

 Lunge Pose with Arms Up

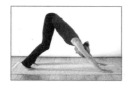 Downward-Facing Dog Pose (Adho Mukha Svanasana)

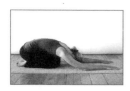 Child's Pose (Adho Mukha Virasana)

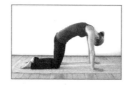 Cat's Pose (Marjaryasana) with Leg Lifts

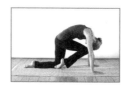 Cat's Pose (Marjaryasana), Knee In

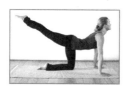 Cat's Pose (Marjaryasana), Leg Extended

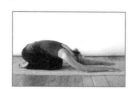 Child's Pose (Adho Mukha Virasana)

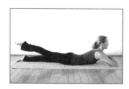 Locust Pose (Salabhasana)

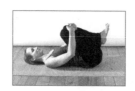 Knees-into-the-Chest Pose (Apanasana)

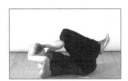

Side-to-Side Abdominal Strengthener

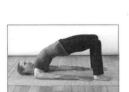

Bridge Pose (Setu Bandha Sarvangasana)

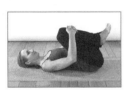

Knees-into-the-Chest Pose (Apanasana)

YIN POSES

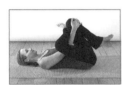

Eye-of-the-Needle Pose

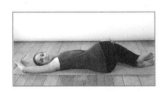

Lying Spinal Twist Pose

Happy Baby Pose/Stirrup Pose

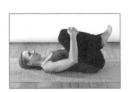

Knees-into-the-Chest Pose

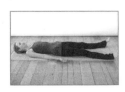

Corpse Pose (Savasana)

Yang Poses

Child's Pose (Adho Mukha Virasana)

Start on your hands and knees. Sit back by moving your hips toward your feet, your knees slightly apart, and your head relaxing toward the floor (Fig. 17.1).

Hold the pose for 5 breaths, centering your attention on the length and depth of each breath as you release any tensions you can sense in your body.

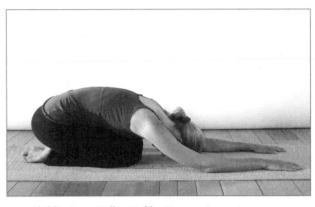

17.1. Child's Pose (Adho Mukha Virasana)

Ruddy Goose (Cakravakasana)

With your hands extended in front of you in Child's Pose, and on an inhalation, slowly come forward onto all fours until your shoulders are above your hands and your hips are above your knees. Lift your shoulders away from your wrists and draw them down your back (Fig. 17.2). On an exhalation, draw your tailbone toward the floor as you move back (Fig. 17.3), allowing your lower back to round but keeping your upper back neutral, ending in Child's Pose (Adho Mukha Virasana; Fig. 17.4). Repeat this back-and-forth movement 5 times, synchronizing the movements exactly with the length of your breaths, about five seconds each.

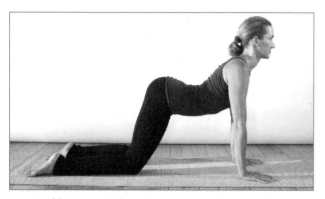

17.2. Ruddy Goose (Cakravakasana), Moving Forward

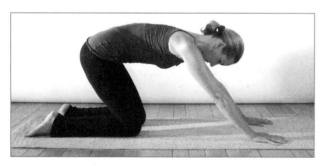

17.3. Ruddy Goose Pose (Cakravakasana), Moving Backward

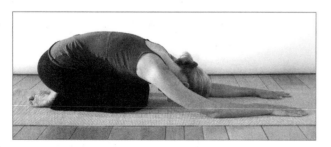

17.4. Child's Pose (Adho Mukha Virasana)

Lunge Pose with Hands Down

The next time you come forward, bring your left foot forward as well until it is under your knee in a lunge (Fig. 17.5). Allow your hips to dip toward the floor as you distribute the bulk of your weight into your left foot. Also allow an even distribution of weight in both hands where they rest on either side of your foot, while also weighting the back leg. Allow your chest to lift and your shoulder blades to drop down your back. Engage the right buttock muscle. Rest the top of your right foot on the floor. Your right knee should feel unburdened, but if you feel uncomfortable because your kneecap (patella) is weighted into the floor, then pull your right leg forward a little, so your weight is not right on the bone but on the soft tissue of the thigh. If it still feels painful, place extra padding under your knee.

Stay here for 5 breaths, bringing your attention to your inner right thigh area while beginning to breathe into your edge, imagining your breath stroking the inner leg as it is stretched. On an exhalation, pull your left foot back and return to Child's Pose (Adho Mukha Virasana). On an inhalation bring the right foot forward and lunge on this side.

Repeat this 5 times.

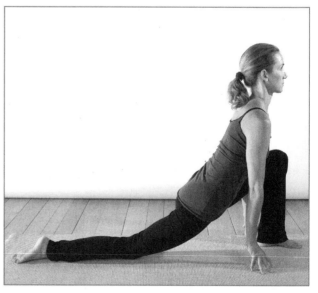

17.5. Lunge Pose with Hands Down

Lunge Pose with Arms Up

Come out of Child's Pose (Adho Mukha Virasana) into another lunge with your left foot forward and settle into it as before, allowing your hips to draw as far forward toward the floor as feels interesting without being alarming. This is the time to develop your skill for recognizing an appropriate edge (not neutral, but not overly intense either). On an inhalation, raise your arms above your head until your hands are shoulder-width apart and facing each other (Fig. 17.6). Maintain the feeling of drawing your hips toward the floor while "hugging" your inner thighs toward each other (while still engaging the right buttock). Ground down through your inner left foot and your right toes, and feel as though your tailbone is directed toward your pubic bone. Lengthen upward along the sides of your body as if your shoulders begin at your waist; allow them to remain broad across your back. Hold this pose for 5 breaths.

You can begin to feel the concept of lines of energy while in this pose. After you have attended to your alignment and can comfortably maintain a slow Ujjayi breath, begin to imagine a tunnel of energy pulsing up your spine and out the crown of your head and fingertips, as well as a counterforce

drawing down into the floor through your tailbone. Allow this radiating energy to influence the lengthening and widening of your body, breath by breath.

On the fifth exhalation, lower your arms and bring your hands to the floor. Inhale as you bring your left foot back, and exhale back to Child's Pose (Adho Mukha Virasana). Repeat the same pose with your right foot forward.

Downward-Facing Dog Pose (Adho Mukha Svanasana)

From Child's Pose (Adho Mukha Virasana), inhale and come forward onto all fours. Tuck your toes under, and as you exhale, lift off your knees and draw your weight back into your legs (Fig. 17.7). (Note: Downward-Facing Dog is often taught with straight legs, but I suggest you start with bent knees [Fig. 17.8] in order to lengthen the lower back and more easily lift the sitting bones. If you have long hamstrings and can easily lift the sitting bones, then practice this pose with straight legs instead.) Continue to lengthen your

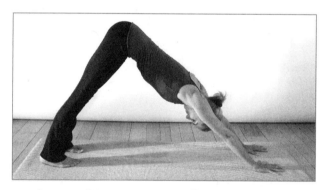

17.7. Downward-Facing Dog Pose (Adho Mukha Svanasana)

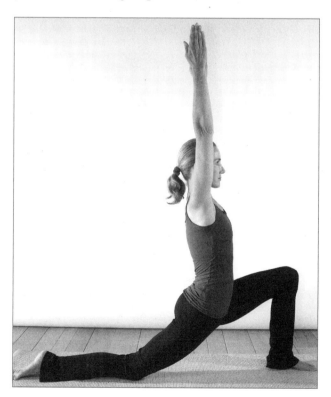

17.6. Lunge Pose with Arms Up

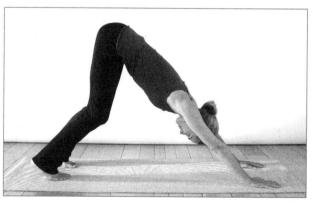

17.8. Downward-Facing Dog Pose (Adho Mukha Svanasana), Variation

arms as you press your hands into the floor with fingers spread. Keep the base of your neck broad and lift your sitting bones up and back, spreading them away from each other. Stay in this pose for 3 to 5 breaths. Exhale and come down into Child's Pose (Adho Mukha Virasana). Rest in Child's Pose for a few breaths.

Floor Sun Salutation (Surya Namaskar) with Downward-Facing Dog Pose (Adho Mukha Svanasana)

Begin with inhaling forward onto all fours and exhaling back as you did earlier (Figs. 17.9 and 17.10).

From Child's Pose (Adho Mukha Virasana), inhale and come up onto your knees with your hands reaching out to the sides and up over your head (Fig. 17.11). As you exhale, bend your arms and bring your shoulder blades down your back as you pull your elbows down and back and spread your fingers. Allow your weight to sit lower as you arch your back, coming about halfway down toward a sitting position (Fig. 17.12). Inhale and draw your hips back up over your knees; lift your arms straight over your head again (Fig. 17.13). Exhale and ease back toward your feet, sweeping your hands to the sides and

down (Fig. 17.14), gradually lowering your head and bringing your hands down as you rest to the floor, sliding your hands in front of you again in Child's Pose (Adho Mukha Virasana; Fig. 17.15) once you are down.

Inhale and raise up, stepping your right foot forward into a lunge (Fig. 17.16). Exhale as you rest the top of your left foot on the floor and lower your hips. Stay for 5 breaths. Inhale and take your right knee back next to the left. Exhale back into Child's Pose (Adho Mukha Virasana; Fig. 17.17).

Inhale and repeat the same kind of lunge on the left side (Fig. 17.18). Rest your back foot down and stay for 5 breaths. Inhale as you bring the left knee back to meet the right, then exhale into Child's Pose (Adho Mukha Virasana).

From Child's Pose, inhale and come forward onto all fours (Fig. 17.19), then exhale as you lift off your knees into Downward-Facing Dog with bent knees (Adho Mukha Svanasana; Fig. 17.20). Inhale as you lengthen your torso and lift your sitting bones, then exhale back into Child's Pose (Adho Mukha Virasana; Fig. 17.21).

You have now completed one full round of Floor Sun Salutation (Surya Namaskar). Repeat the whole process 2 to 3 more times, then rest in Child's Pose (Adho Mukha Virasana).

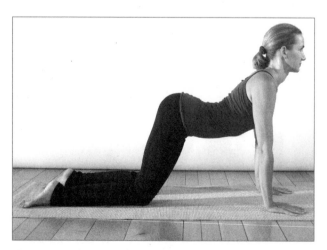

17.9. Floor Sun Salutation / Ruddy Goose Pose (Cakravakasana), Moving Forward

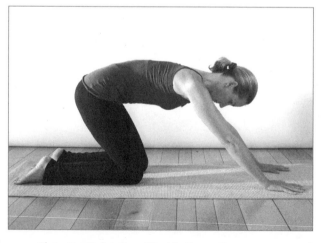

17.10. Floor Sun Salutation / Ruddy Goose Pose (Cakravakasana), Moving Backward

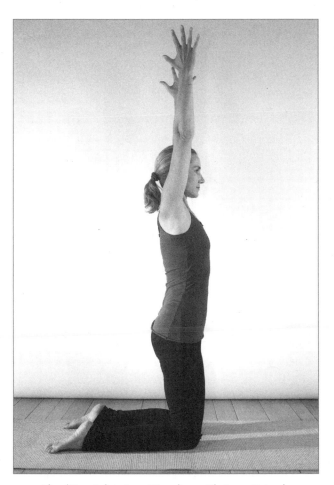

17.11. Floor Sun Salutation / Kneeling with Arms Raised

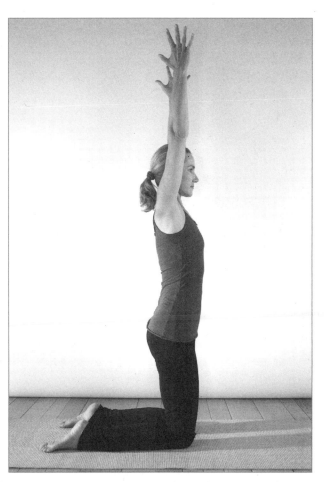

17.13. Floor Sun Salutation / Kneeling with Arms Raised

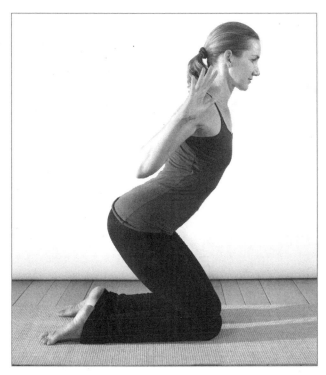

17.12. Floor Sun Salutation / Kneeling Halfway with Arms Bent

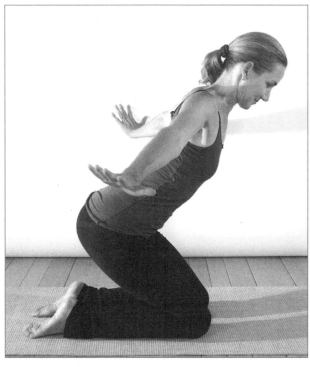

17.14. Floor Sun Salutation / Lowering with Arms to the Sides

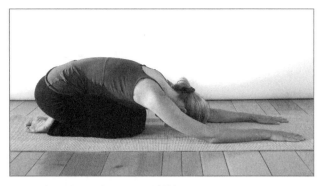

17.15. Floor Sun Salutation / Child's Pose
(Adho Mukha Virasana)

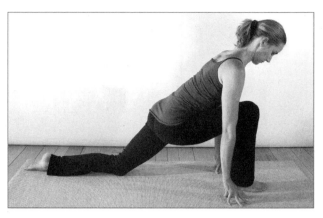

17.16. Floor Sun Salutation / Lunge with Right Foot Forward

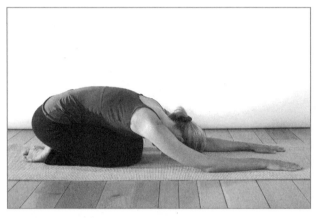

17.17. Floor Sun Salutation / Child's Pose (Adho Mukha Virasana)

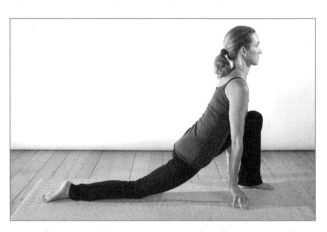

17.18. Floor Sun Salutation / Lunge with Left Foot Forward

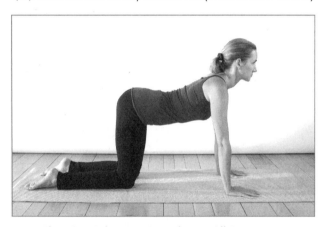

17.19. Floor Sun Salutation / Kneeling on All Fours

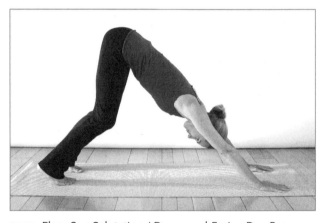

17.20. Floor Sun Salutation / Downward-Facing Dog Pose
(Adho Mukha Svanasana)

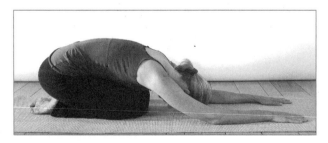

17.21. Floor Sun Salutation / Child's Pose
(Adho Mukha Virasana)

Cat's Pose (Marjaryasana) with Leg Lifts

From Child's Pose (Adho Mukha Virasana), inhale and come up onto all fours. Spread your fingers wide and press your whole hand into the floor while dropping your head and rounding your back, like a cat yawning. As you inhale, start to lift your sitting bones, arch your spine, lengthening the front of your body, while lifting your chin up (Fig. 17.22). Exhale and reverse the arch by drawing your tailbone under, rounding your whole back, and dropping your head (Fig. 17.23). Repeat this movement for 5 breaths.

On the sixth exhalation, while you are rounding your back, bring your right knee in toward your head, while lengthening your arms and pressing down through your hands (Fig. 17.24). As you inhale, arch your back and send your right leg behind you as you straighten it, spreading your toes as you lift the leg up and back (Fig. 17.25). Be aware of how easy it is to lift your hip with your leg; keep your right hip level with the left and only lift your leg as high as it can go without lifting your hip as well.

Exhale and bring your knee back in toward your head, pointing your toes so your foot does not touch the floor. Repeat this movement for 5 breaths.

Switch sides and repeat the leg lifts for another 5 breaths.

Exhale back into Child's Pose (Adho Mukha Virasana) and rest for a few breaths.

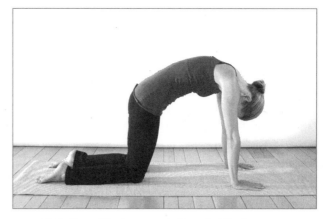

17.23. Cat's Pose (Marjaryasana), Rounded Back

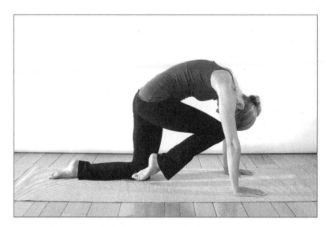

17.24. Cat's Pose (Marjaryasana), Knee In

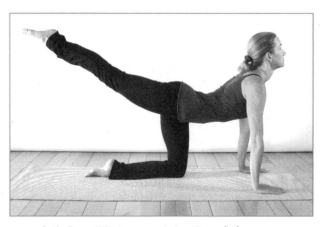

17.25. Cat's Pose (Marjaryasana), Leg Extended

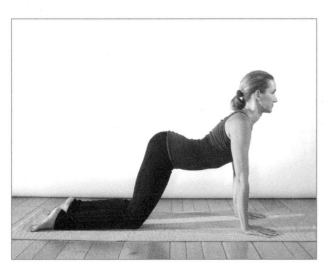

17.22. Cat's Pose (Marjaryasana), Arched Back

Locust Pose (Salabhasana)

Lie on your belly with your legs outstretched and your arms in front of you, your hands around your elbows; rest your head on your forearms. Draw your pubic bone toward the floor, and as you inhale, lift your head, chest, and right leg off the floor, spreading your toes and keeping your knee straight (Fig. 17.26). Exhale and return to your starting position.

Inhale and repeat, but lift your left leg this time. Exhale and lower back to the floor to complete the first round. If you have any pain in your lower back, keep both legs on the floor as you raise your head and chest (Fig. 17.27). Do 4 more rounds. Rest on your belly for a few breaths, then roll over onto your back.

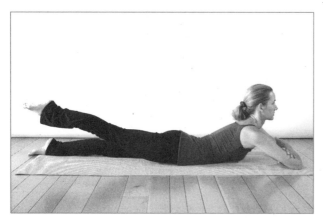

17.26. Locust Pose (Salabhasana)

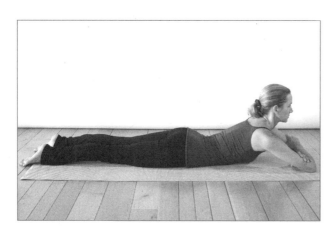

17.27. Locust Pose (Salabhasana), Variation

Side-to-Side Abdominal Strengthener

Place both hands behind your head and interlace your fingers while bringing your knees into your chest. Inhale, then as you exhale, draw your left elbow toward the outside of your right knee (Fig. 17.28). Try not to lean all the way onto your right shoulder. Inhale and lie back down, spreading your elbows back toward the floor and lengthen-

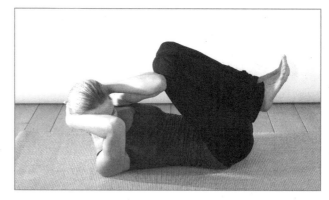

17.28. Side-to-Side Abdominal Strengthener

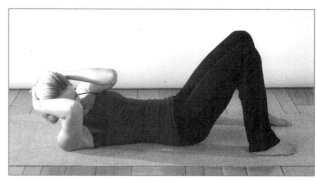

17.29. Side-to-Side Abdominal Strengthener, Variation 1

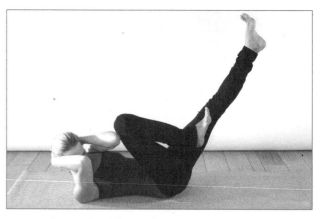

17.30. Side-to-Side Abdominal Strengthener, Variation 2

ing your abdominals. On the next exhalation, take your right elbow toward the outside of your left knee, again attempting to keep your weight in the center of your back rather than leaning onto your left shoulder. Repeat this for 5 breaths on each side. If you have a weak or sensitive back, keep your feet on the ground instead, with the knees bent. Press your lower back into the floor and continue with the same instructions from above (Fig. 17.29). If you have a strong back and want to intensify this pose, extend the left leg out as you are going over to the right, and the right leg out as you bring your elbows over to the left. Be sure to press the lower back into the floor throughout this pose (Fig. 17.30).

Bridge Pose (Setu Bandha Sarvangasana)

Lie on your back, bend your knees, and place your feet under them hip-width apart. Spread your toes and feel the floor under both feet. Let your hands rest on the floor beside your hips, and keep the weight of your head centered evenly, with your chin in line with the center of your chest and your forehead on about the same plane as your chin. Exhale and draw your belly down, flattening your lower back into the floor. Inhale and press your weight into both feet evenly; draw your hips up toward the sky as high as they are willing to go without a strain (Fig. 17.31). As you exhale, with your tailbone drawn in toward your pubic bone, round your spine down to the floor, vertebra by vertebra. Repeat this lifting and lowering 5 times.

On the fifth inhalation, draw your arms over your head on the ground and lift your hips as before. Stay in this position for 5 breaths. On each inhalation, extend out through your spine and arms, and with each exhalation, press your feet a little more firmly into the floor and feel your hips rising. Imagine that you have a soft, hip-width block between your legs and that you are keeping it in place by hugging your inner thighs around it. This will help you engage the adductor muscles along your inner thighs, which help support your lower back and hips. On the fifth exhalation, lower back to the floor, vertebra by vertebra, beginning at your neck.

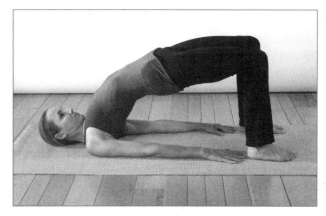

17.31. Bridge Pose (Setu Bandha Sarvangasana)

Knees-into-the-Chest Pose (Apanasana)

While lying on your back with your head resting comfortably, bring both knees into your chest and interlace your fingers around your upper shins (Fig. 17.32). You can hold one end of a strap in each hand and loop this over your shins if you cannot bring your hands together.

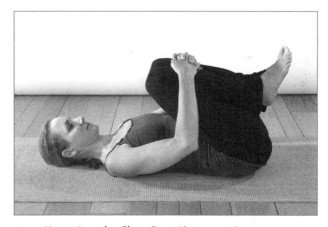

17.32. Knees-into-the-Chest Pose (Apanasana)

Yin Poses

Eye-of-the-Needle Pose

Lie on your back with your feet on the floor and your knees bent; place your right ankle on top of your left knee. Draw your left knee toward your chest, reach your hands around your shins, and interlace your fingers (Fig. 17.33). Your left arm reaches around the outside of your left leg, and your right arm is between your legs. As you draw your knee toward you, keep your sacrum on the floor, and your shoulders and head on the floor. If you cannot clasp your hands easily, you can hold a strap between your hands, and/or place a small blanket under your head so that your chin and forehead rest at the same height. You can also do this pose against the wall as described on page 63. Relax your left ankle and close your eyes while you remain in this pose for 3 to 5 minutes.

You will feel sensations in your right hip intensifying over time, meaning the pose is stimulating the Liver and Spleen meridians in your inner groin area as well as the Gallbladder meridian along your outer right hip. (These meridians are discussed in detail in chapters 8 and 10.)

Exhale as you release your hands and rest with both feet on the floor, allowing your knees to drop in toward each other for a minute or so before repeating the same pose on the other side.

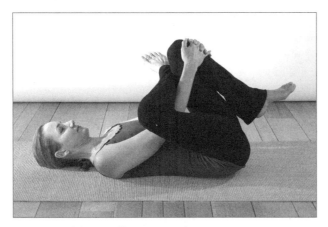

17.33. Eye-of-the-Needle Pose

Lying Spinal Twist Pose (Jathara Parivatanasana)

Do Lying Spinal Twist Pose (Fig. 17.34) as described on page 51.

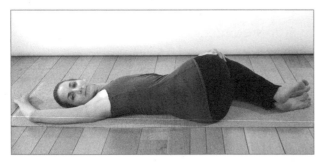

17.34. Lying Spinal Twist Pose

Stirrup Pose

Do Stirrup Pose (Fig. 17.35) or its variation (Fig. 17.36) as described on page 53.

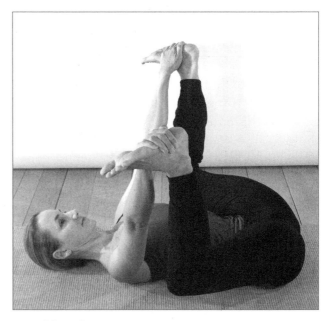

17.35. Stirrup Pose

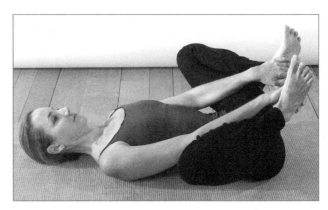

17.36. Stirrup Pose, Variation

Corpse Pose (Savasana)

Come into Corpse Pose (Fig. 17.37) as described on page 47.

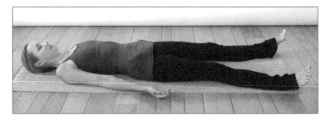

17.37. Corpse Pose

Sun Salutation (Surya Namaskar) Yang Practice

This simple, well-rounded practice brings length and strength to all the core muscles in the torso. I love it as a short but dynamic complement to a long Yin session and to breed stability and warmth through the whole system. There is a natural cyclical feeling in going through the series and coming back to Mountain Pose (Tadasana) that engenders a sense of coordination and competency through slow, strong, and conscious movements.

 Mountain Pose (Tadasana)

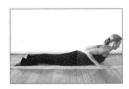 Cobra Pose (Bhujangasana)

 Standing Forward Bend (Uttanasana)

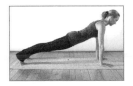 Plank Pose (Phalakasana)

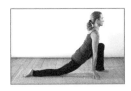 Low Lunge Pose (Anjaneyasana)

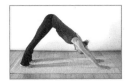 Downward-Facing Dog Pose (Adho Mukha Svanasana)

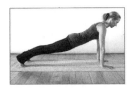 Plank Pose (Phalakasana)

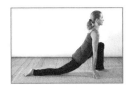 Low Lunge Pose (Anjaneyasana) (right foot forward)

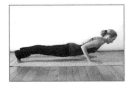 Four-Limbed Staff Pose (Chaturanga Dandasana)

 Standing Forward Bend (Uttanasana)

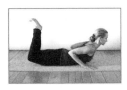 Bow Pose (Dhanurasana)

 Mountain Pose (Tadasana)

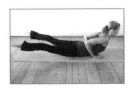 Locust Pose (Salabhasana)

Mountain Pose (Tadasana)

Begin by standing with your feet together and your toes spread. Lift your kneecaps and stack the hips above the ankles. Elongate your side waist, lift your chest, and relax the front ribs down. Draw your shoulders down your back while lengthening up through the crown of your head. Take 5 breaths.

Inhale and raise your arms to the sides until your hands face each other, shoulder-width apart.

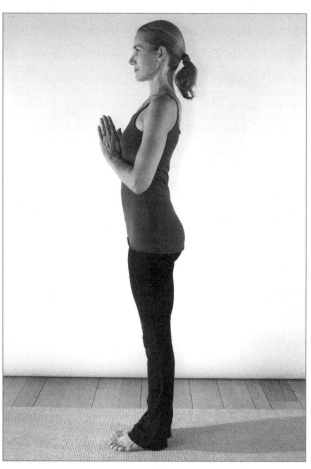

17.38. Mountain Pose (Tadasana)

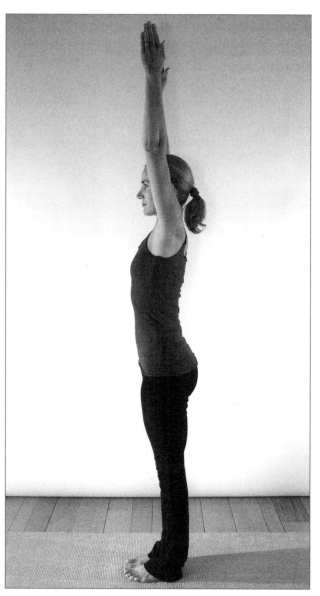

17.39. Mountain Pose (Tadasana) with Arms Overhead

Standing Forward Bend (Uttanasana)

Exhale and draw both groins back as you bring your arms down and fold forward (Fig. 17.40).

Standing Forward Bend (Uttanasana) with Chest Lifted

Inhale and lift the chest as you come up on the fingertips, drawing your shoulders away from the ears and spreading the sitting bones (Fig. 17.41).

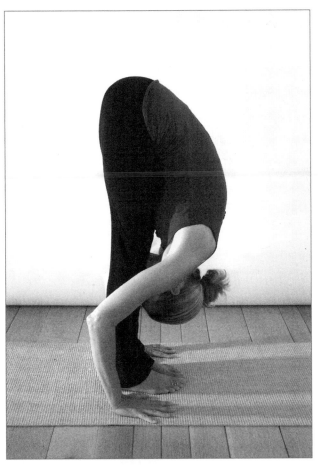

17.40. Standing Forward Bend (Uttanasana)

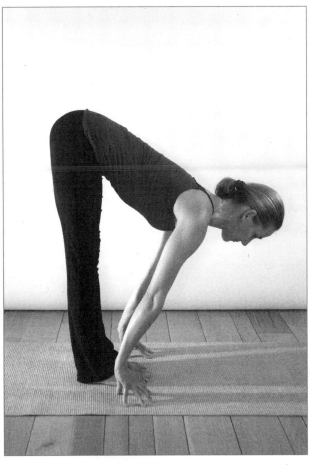

17.41. Standing Forward Bend (Uttanasana) with Chest Lifted

Low Lunge Pose (Anjaneyasana)

On an exhalation, step back to a low lunge with the right foot (Fig. 17.42). Stay for 5 breaths with your hands beside the feet, or reach up with the hands parallel and shoulder-width apart (Fig. 17.43).

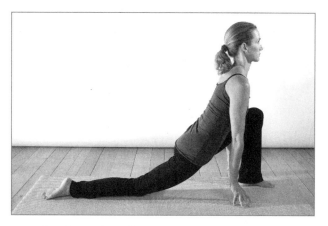

17.42. Low Lunge Pose (Anjaneyasana)

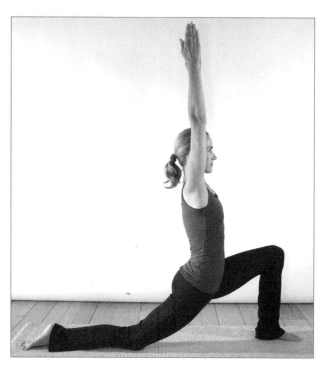

17.43. Low Lunge Pose (Anjaneyasana) with Arms Overhead

Plank Pose (Phalakasana)

As you inhale, place your weight evenly onto both hands as you step the left foot back to meet the right in Plank Pose (Phalakasana; Fig. 17.44). With both arms straight and the hands directly under the shoulders, draw your navel toward your spine and your tailbone slightly in. The legs can be strong and straight, or the knees can rest down on the floor (Fig. 17.45).

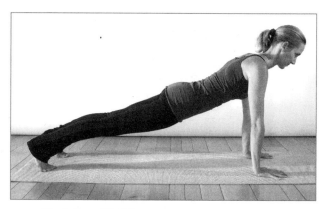

17.44. Plank Pose (Phalakasana)

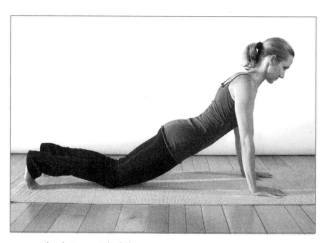

17.45. Plank Pose (Phalakasana), Variation

Four-Limbed Staff Pose (Chaturanga Dandasana)

As you exhale—(with either the legs straight (Fig. 17.46) or the knees on the floor (Fig. 17.47) if this is too difficult)—bend the elbows and, keeping the shoulders drawn down away from the ears and your navel drawn back, slowly lower the torso and legs into the Four-Limbed Staff Pose. Simultaneously actively engaging the arm muscles (deltoids and triceps), the abdominal muscles, and the inner legs (the abductors). Inhale and straighten the arms into Plank Pose again (Fig. 17.44) and repeat, bending and straightening the arms for 3 to 5 breaths. On the last exhalation, lower all the way down (Fig. 17.48).

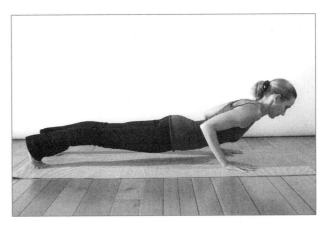

17.46. Four-Limbed Staff Pose (Chaturanga Dandasana)

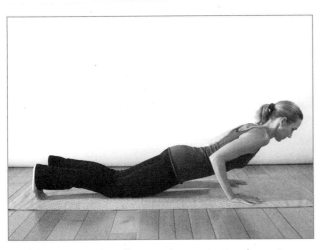

17.47. Four-Limbed Staff Pose (Chaturanga Dandasana), Variation

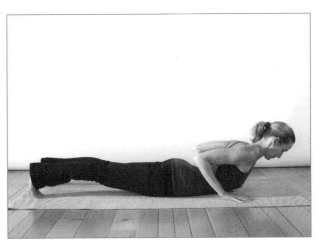

17.48. Four-Limbed Staff Pose (Chaturanga Dandasana), Floor Variation

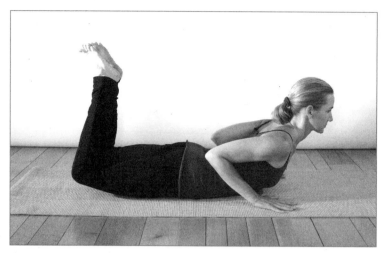

17.49. Bow Pose (Dhanurasana)

Bow Pose (Dhanurasana)

Inhale and bend the knees. Rest the feet together as you push down through the hands and pubic bone, lift the head, chest, and thighs, while spreading the toes. Keep the elbows squeezing in near your ribs and hug the inner thighs (they need not be together, though) (Fig. 17.49). Stay for 3 to 5 breaths.

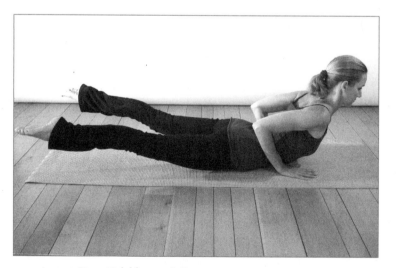

17.50. Locust Pose (Salabhasana), Part 1

Locust Pose (Salabhasana)

On the 3rd or 5th exhalation, straighten the legs in Locust Pose (Salabhasana) (Fig. 17.50). The upper body is primarily the same as bow pose, but with the legs straight. Inhale, lift the chest a bit more, and widen the legs (Fig. 17.51). Exhale, bring the legs together, keeping the hands down, the elbows in, and the chest and legs lifted. (Although the head is lifted, drop the chin down slightly.) Take 3 to 5 breaths moving the legs apart as you inhale and bringing them back together as you exhale. On the fifth exhalation, lower down (Fig. 17.48).

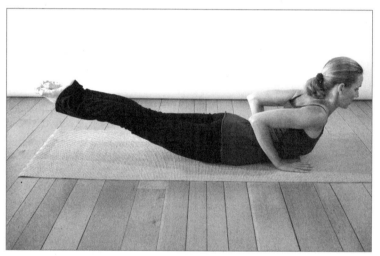

17.51. Locust Pose (Salabhasana), Part 2

Cobra Pose (Bhujangasana)

Keeping the chest and head in the same lifted position as Locust Pose, the fingers spread and the legs down, inhale and widen across the chest as you lift up the breast bone while keeping the ribs touching the floor (Fig. 17.52). Draw the shoulders down the back, bringing the elbows in and lifting the kneecaps. You can also lift the ribs while keeping the navel down for a slightly deeper backbend (Fig. 17.53). This is a medium height for Cobra Pose. The highest lift in Cobra occurs when you lift the front body completely up, except for the lower belly and pubic bone (Fig. 17.54). Remember to continue to draw the chest forward while the shoulders go back; the top of the sternum lifts while the pubic bone and legs descend. The inner thighs hug inward while the chest and collar bones widen. Stay for 3 to 5 breaths.

Plank Pose (Phalakasana)

Inhale and lift up to Plank Pose (Phalakasana; Fig. 17.55), as described on page 128.

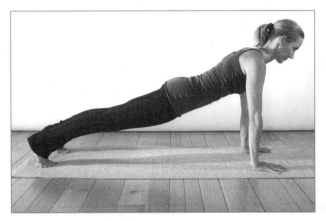

17.55. Plank Pose (Phalakasana)

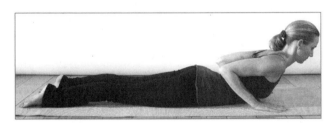

17.52. Cobra Pose (Bhujangasana), Part 1

Downward-Facing Dog Pose (Adho Mukha Svanasana)

Exhale as you draw the hips back into Downward-Facing Dog Pose (Adho Mukha Svanasana; Fig. 17.56), as described on page 117. Stay for 5 breaths.

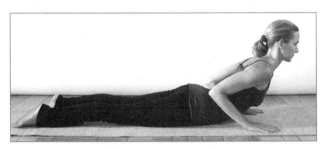

17.53. Cobra Pose (Bhujangasana), Part 2

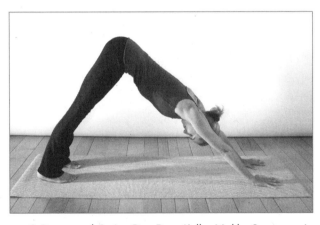

17.56. Downward-Facing Dog Pose (Adho Mukha Svanasana)

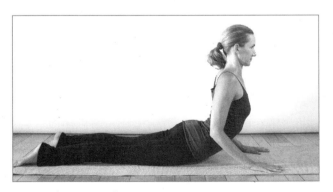

17.54. Cobra Pose (Bhujangasana), Part 3

Low Lunge Pose (Anjaneyasana)

On an inhalation, step the right foot forward into Low Lunge Pose (Anjaneyasana; Fig. 17.57), as described at the beginning of this sequence. Exhale, and lower the back leg into a low lunge. Inhale, raise the arms, and stay for 3 to 5 breaths (Fig. 17.58).

Standing Forward Bend (Uttanasana)

On an exhalation, bring your hands down to the floor. Inhale, and step your back foot forward, so your feet are together. Lift your chest as described on page 127 (Fig. 17.59). Exhale and fold forward in Standing Forward Bend (Uttanasana; Fig. 17.60). Stay in the pose for 3 to 5 breaths.

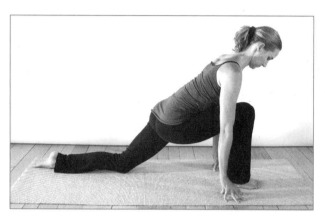

17.57. Low Lunge Pose (Anjaneyasana)

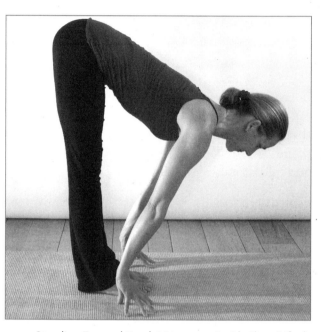

17.59. Standing Forward Bend (Uttanasana) with Chest Lifted

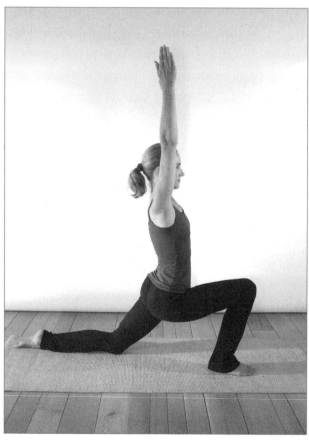

17.58. Low Lunge Pose (Anjaneyasana) with Arms Overhead

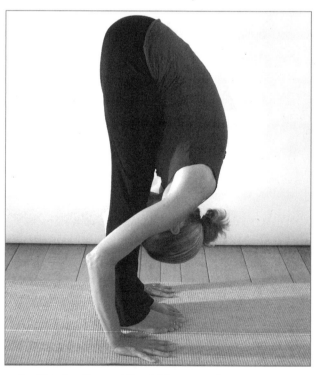

17.60. Standing Forward Bend (Uttanasana)

Mountain Pose (Tadasana)

On an inhalation, come all the way up into Mountain Pose (Tadasana) and raise your arms overhead (Fig. 17.61), as described on page 126. Exhale and lower your arms to your sides (Fig. 17.62).

This combination of poses lengthens and strengthens all the major muscles along the center of the body, including the trapezius (shoulder muscles), the pectoralis (chest muscles), the serratus and latissimus muscles of the sides and back, the hamstring, quadricep, and adductor muscles in the legs.

Repeat this sun salutation cycle at least 3 to 5 more times. I have listed some variations below during the lunge poses that will allow you to emphasize slightly different areas in your body in each one. The variations listed below are possible in each lunge. Stay 5 to 10 breaths on each side.

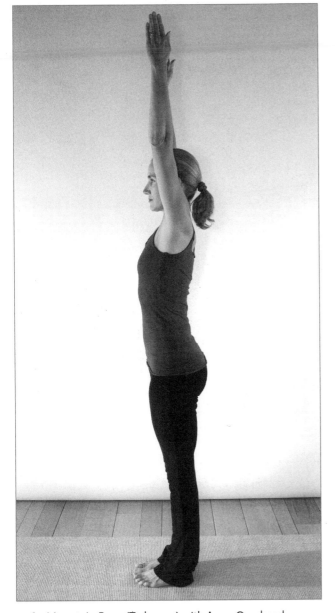

17.61. Mountain Pose (Tadasana) with Arms Overhead

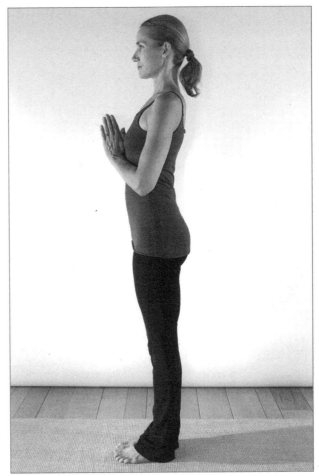

17.62. Mountain Pose (Tadasana)

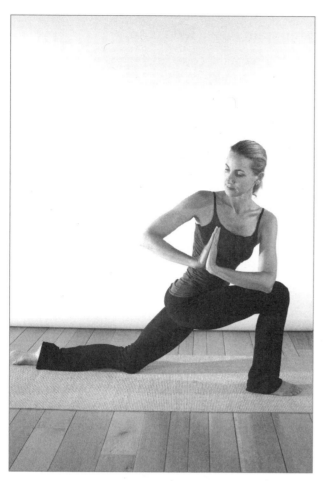

17.63. Lunge Pose with Twist (Anjaneyasana Variation)

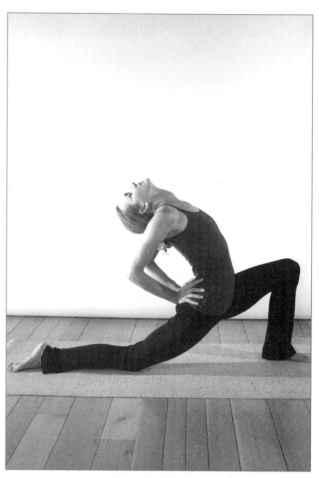

17.64. Lunge Pose with Backbend (Anjaneyasana variation)

Round Two—Lunge twist

Follow the same instructions for Lunge Pose but on an inhale bring the hands together in front of the chest. As you exhale, bring your right elbow over to rest on the outside of the left thigh. As you press the hands toward each other lift the chest while turning your torso to the left (Fig. 17.63 shows twisting to the right). Keep the interior of the left foot grounded, the right buttock engaged, and the right shoulder down the back. Continue to hug the inner thigh in. Stay 3 to 5 breaths. Exhale, release the hands, and bring them to the floor and continue with the sequence. (This twisting lunge will emphasize lengthening the rhomboids between the shoulders as well as utilizing all the muscles, both front and back, in your torso while creating a massaging effect on the inner organs.)

Round Three—Lunge backbend

Follow the same instructions for Lunge Pose but on an inhale bring the hands back on the buttocks with the fingers facing up. Keep the elbows in and lift the chest, lengthening the side waist while weighting the hips down. Keep the right buttock engaged and press down through the inner left foot and all the back toes. (This pose will further lengthen the muscles in the front body, including the pectoralis and abdominals, as well as strengthening the back body, including the latissimus, the erector spinae, and the trapezius. Note: if you have sensitivities in your neck, do not lay your head back; instead keep it upright and look straight ahead.)

Round Four—Lunge with the back foot toward the buttocks

Follow the same instructions for Lunge Pose but on an inhale reach for your right foot, slowly bringing it in toward your right buttock (Fig. 17.65). Continue to draw the inner thighs toward each other, keeping the right buttock engaged and the toes spread. *Do not force the foot in,* but imagine the breath to be slowly drawn across the top thigh of the right leg and stay 3 to 5 breaths. (This variation will further lengthen the quadriceps, i.e., the front thigh muscles.)

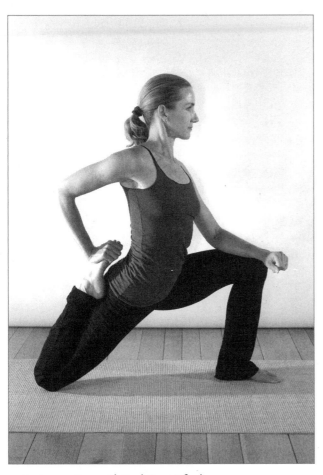

17.65. Lunge Pose with Back Foot Lifted (Anjaneyasana variation)

Round Five—Lunge wide or Hanumanasana (splits)

Follow the same instructions for Lunge Pose but on an inhale move the left foot further forward than the knee, place your hands on the floor (or on blocks), and continue to hug the inner thighs together, keeping the right buttock engaged and allowing the hip to weight down while the chest lifts up (Fig. 17.66). If you can move the foot way forward, rest the left calf and back of the thigh down in splits while keeping the right top of the thigh on the floor and the right hip coming forward (Fig.17.67). (Both of these lunge variations further stretch the inner legs—i.e., the adductors—and deep hip muscles, i.e., the psoas.) To come out, inhale and draw the left foot back using your abdominals. Continue with Plank Pose.

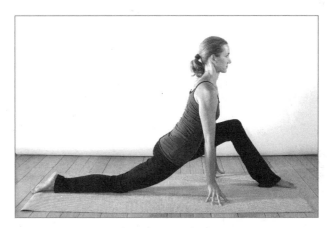

17.66. Lunge Pose with Wide Legs (Anjaneyasana variation)

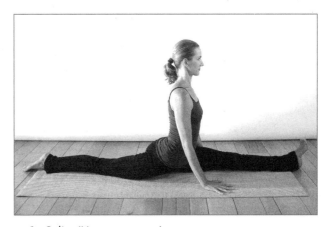

17.67. Splits (Hanumanasana)

Practice for Stimulating the Kidneys and Circulating Yang Chi to the Core

Sun Salutation
(Surya Namaskar)
with Lunges (see page 125 sequence)

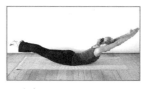 Locust Pose, Part 2

 Chair Pose (Utkatasana)

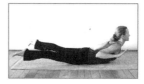 Locust Pose, Part 3

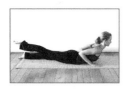 Locust Pose (Salabhasana)
(with one leg lifted)

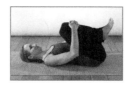 Knees-into-the-Chest Pose
(Apanasana)

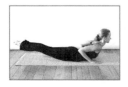 Locust Pose (Salabhasana)
(with both legs lifted)

 Bridge Pose
(Setu Bandha Sarvangasana)
(with leg raised)

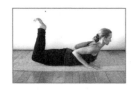 Bow Pose (Dhanurasana)
(with the hands on the floor)

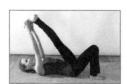 Lying One-Legged Forward
Bend
(Supta Padangusthasana)

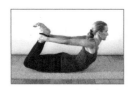 Bow Pose (Dhanurasana)
(holding the ankles)

 Lying One-Legged Forward Bend
(Supta Padangusthasana) Variation 1

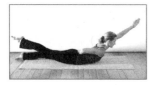 Locust Pose
(Salabhasana), Part 1

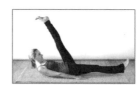 Variation 2

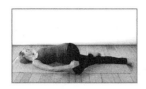 Lying Spinal Twist Pose (Jathara Parivatanasana)

 Lying Straddle Splits (Supta Konasana)

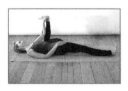 Half-Stirrup Pose (Ardha Ananda Balasana)

 Lying Straddle Splits (Supta Konasana), Part 2

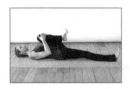 One-Knee-into-the-Chest Pose (Ardha Apanasana)

 Lying Straddle Splits (Supta Konasana), Part 3

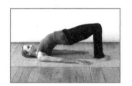 Bridge Pose (Setu Bandha Sarvangasana) (feet and knees together)

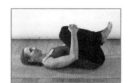 Knees-into-the-Chest Pose (Apanasana)

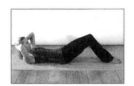 Abdominal/Sacral Strengthener

 Inverted Action Pose or Beginners' Shoulderstand (Viparita Karani) with variations

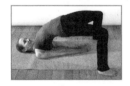 Bridge Pose (Setu Bandha Sarvangasana) (feet and knees wide apart)

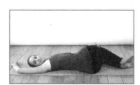 Lying Spinal Twist Pose (Jathara Parivatanasana)

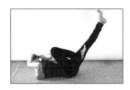 Opposite Leg Abdominal Strengthener

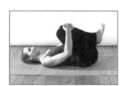 Knees-into-the-Chest Pose (Apanasana)

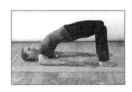 Bridge Pose (Setu Bandha Sarvangasana) (feet hip-width apart)

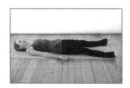 Corpse Pose (Savasana)

Sun Salutation (Surya Namaskar) with Lunges

Do the entire sequence from page 125. Complete 1 to 5 rounds before proceeding to the next pose.

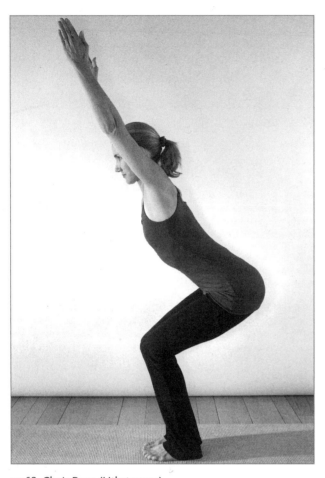

17.68. Chair Pose (Utkatasana)

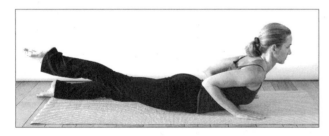

17.69. Locust Pose (Salabhasana) with One Leg Lifted

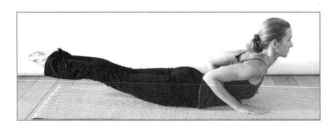

17.70. Locust Pose (Salabhasana) with Both Legs Lifted

Chair Pose (Utkatasana)

From Mountain Pose (Tadasana), inhale and raise your arms overhead. As you exhale, bend your knees into a squat and arch your lower back slightly (Fig. 17.68). Be sure not to tuck your sitting bones under; instead, draw them toward the back of your mat. This will protect and strengthen your lower back. Keep the arms shoulder-width apart, the head centered, and the knees hugging each other. Stay here for 6 to 8 breaths.

Exhale and come down into a standing forward bend, inhale, lift the chest, exhale, step the right foot back, and inhale as you step the left foot back so you are in Plank Pose. Exhale as you lower to the push-up position before resting on your belly.

Locust Pose (Salabhasana)

Lie on your belly with your hands resting under the chest. Inhale and lift your head and chest along with your right leg (Fig. 17.69). Extend energy out through your right foot and spread your toes, keeping your right leg rotated slightly inward. Your left leg can also be active if you lift your kneecap but keep your foot on the floor.

Exhale and bring your right leg down as you rest your head down. Inhale and repeat with your left leg, completing 1 round. Do 3 to 5 rounds.

Next, inhale and lift your head, chest, and both legs off the floor (Fig. 17.70). Press your feet away from you while spreading your toes and rotating your legs slightly inward. Stay up for 3 to 5 breaths. Exhale and come down. Repeat for 1 to 3 rounds.

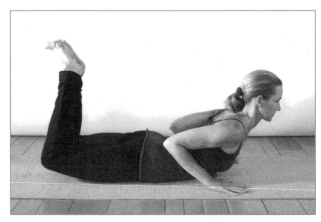

17.71 Bow Pose (Dhanurasana) with Hands on the Floor

Bow Pose (Dhanurasana) (with the hands on the floor)

Lie on your belly with your hands next to your chest and your elbows beside your ribs. Bend your knees and allow your feet to touch. Bring your tailbone toward the floor, and as you inhale, lift your head, chest, and both legs toward the ceiling (Fig. 17.71). Stay up for 3 to 5 breaths while engaging your inner thighs. There is no need to lift your chin; instead, allow it to remain on the same (vertical) plane as your forehead.

Exhale and release back to the floor. Repeat 1 to 3 times.

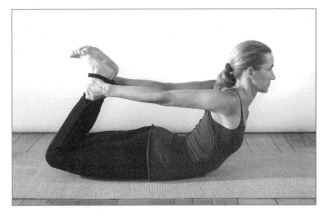

17.72. Bow Pose (Dhanurasana)

Bow Pose (Dhanurasana) (holding the ankles)

Lying on your stomach with your pubic bone dropping down toward the floor, inhale and bring your feet up toward your buttocks, reaching your hands back for your outer ankles. On the next inhalation, keeping your inner thighs engaged, lift your head, chest, and thighs, drawing your weight back toward your pubic bone, rather than forward onto your ribs (Fig. 17.72). Stay in this pose for 3 to 5 breaths. Be careful not to strain in this pose, and only come up as high as you can without losing connection with your breath rhythms.

Exhale and lower your chest and head before slowly letting go of your ankles.

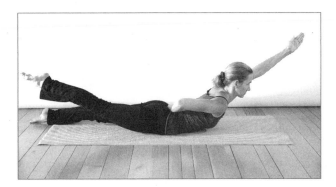

17.73. Locust Pose (Salabhasana), Part 1

Locust Pose (Salabhasana)

Lie on your belly with your hands resting on your sacrum, palms up. Inhale and bring your left arm forward and up as you lift your head, chest, and right leg (Fig. 17.73). Keep your head in line with your raised arm, and draw energy out through your right leg, spreading your toes. As you exhale, bring your left arm back, lower your right leg, and rest your left cheek on the mat. Inhale and raise up again, this time bringing your right arm around and up, and lifting your left leg. Exhale and sweep your right arm back, lower your leg, and rest your right cheek on the mat. Repeat 3 to 5 times on each side.

Next, inhale and bring both arms up and forward while lifting both legs and spreading your toes (Fig. 17.74). Keep your head (or ears) aligned

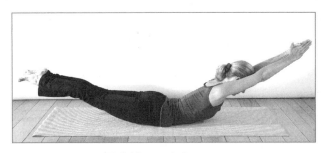

17.74. Locust Pose (Salabhasana), Part 2

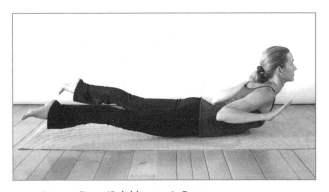

17.75. Locust Pose (Salabhasana), Part 3

with your arms. Exhale and bend your elbows, pulling your hands back and spreading your fingers while widening your legs and spreading your toes (Fig. 17.75). Inhale and straighten your arms, bringing your hands toward each other while drawing your legs back together (keep them lifted). Exhale and repeat—widening your legs, bending your elbows, and keeping your chest up—for 3 to 5 breaths.

When you are ready to come down, exhale and draw your arms back; rest your hands on your sacrum again; and lower your head, chest, and legs.

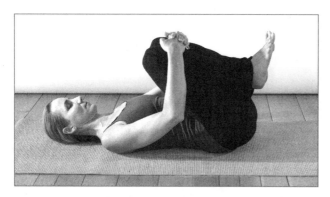

17.76. Knees-into-the-Chest Pose (Apanasana)

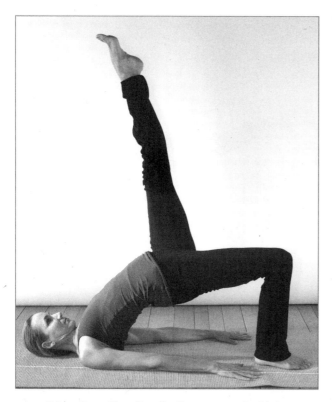

17.77. Bridge Pose (Setu Bandha Sarvangasana) with Leg Raised

Knees-into-the-Chest Pose (Apanasana)

Roll over on your back and bring your knees up to your chest, interlacing your fingers over your shins (Fig. 17.76). Keep your sacrum, shoulders, and chin down. Stay in this pose for 3 to 5 breaths.

Bridge Pose (Setu Bandha Sarvangasana), with Leg Raised

Place both feet on the floor under your knees, hip-width apart. Keep your hands on the floor beside you and lift your left leg straight up above your hips, sending energy up through your foot and spreading your toes. Inhale pushing into the right foot, lift your hips (Fig. 17.77), then exhale and lower back to the floor. Repeat this 6 to 8 times. On the last one, stay up for 6 to 8 breaths, engaging your inner thighs, pressing down through your hands, and lifting up through your hips and chest. Exhale and come down. Keep your leg lifted while going to the next pose.

Lying One-Legged Forward Bend (Supta Padangusthasana)

With your left leg still lifted, reach your hands behind your left thigh, knee, calf, or foot (as shown in Fig. 17.78). (You can also place a strap around the sole of your left foot, holding one end with each hand.) Keeping your sacrum down, press forward through the back of your left knee, away from your head, bringing your leg straight, while at the same time bringing your foot toward your head. Do each of these actions simultaneously while also lengthening your left hip away from the ribs and rotating the leg slightly inward. Stay in this pose for 8 to 10 breaths. On the next inhalation, raise your head and upper back, bringing your forehead toward your left leg (Fig. 17.79). You can also try this same pose with the right leg extended and lifted a few inches from the ground while pressing your lower back into the floor (Fig. 17.80). Stay in this pose for 8 to 10 breaths. Exhale and as you lower your head, bend the left knee into the chest as you proceed to the next pose.

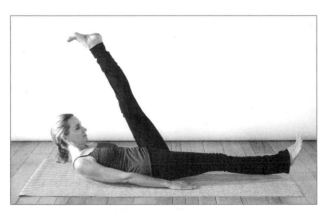

17.78. Lying One-Legged Forward Bend
(Supta Padangusthasana)

Lying Spinal Twist Pose
(Jathara Parivatanasana)

Release your left knee and place your foot on the inside of your right knee. Keeping your right leg straight, twist over to the right side. Straighten your left arm out in line with your shoulder, palm down, turning your head to the left. Keep the back of your left shoulder grounded as you take your left knee over as far as it is willing to go (Fig. 17.81). If your left knee does not rest on the floor, place a cushion under it. Stay in this pose for 8 to 10 breaths. Inhale and bring your knee back to center; continue to the next pose.

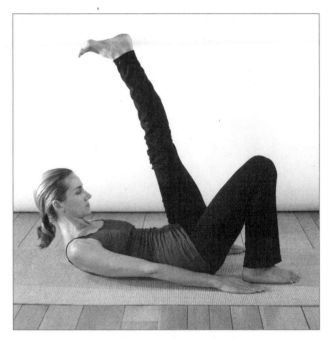

17.79. Lying One-Legged Forward Bend
(Supta Padangusthasana), Variation 1

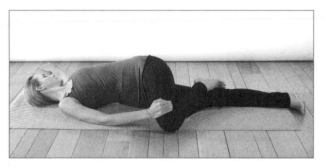

17.81. Lying Spinal Twist Pose (Jathara Parivatanasana)

Half-Stirrup Pose (Ardha Ananda
Balasana)

From your bent-knee position, bring your left foot back over and place your left hand along the sole of your foot, near the arch. Bring the foot above your left knee while keeping your right hip weighted with your right hand (Fig. 17.82). Stay in this pose for 8 to 10 breaths. Exhale and release your left foot as you proceed to the next pose.

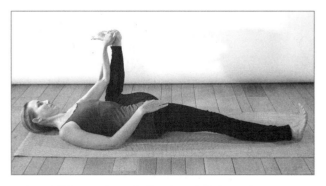

17.80. Lying One-Legged Forward Bend
(Supta Padangusthasana), Variation 2

17.82. Half-Stirrup Pose (Ardha Ananda Balasana)

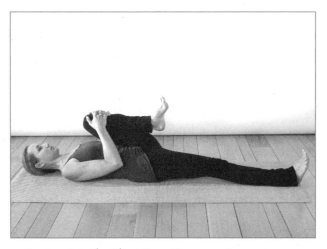

17.83. Knee-into-the-Chest Pose (Apanasana)

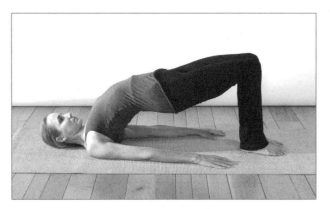

17.84. Bridge Pose (Setu Bandha Sarvangasana), Feet and Knees Together

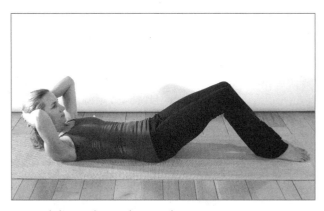

17.85. Abdominal/Sacral Strengthener

One-Knee-into-the-Chest Pose (Ardha Apanasana)

Inhale, and bring your left knee into your chest, interlacing your fingers around the shin (Fig. 17.83). Continue to extend through your right leg, and keep your shoulders drawn down your back. Stay for 6 to 8 breaths. Exhale and place your left foot flat on the floor under your left knee and lift your right leg straight up.

Repeat the last five poses on the right side, starting with Bridge Pose (Setu Bandha Sarvangasana) with the right leg raised.

Bridge Pose (Setu Bandha Sarvangasana)

While lying on your back, bend your knees and bring both feet together, flat on the floor, under your knees. Keep your hands beside you and inhale, lifting your hips and chest (Fig. 17.84). Bring your hips as high as they are willing to go while keeping the inner knees touching, exhale and lower down, rounding your spine back to the floor one vertebra at a time. Repeat this 6 to 8 times. On the last one, stay in the pose for 6 to 8 breaths, then exhale and lower to the floor.

Abdominal/Sacral Strengthener

Still lying on your back with knees bent and feet together, move your feet as far forward as possible without lifting the soles of your feet. Place your hands behind your head. Draw your lower back toward the floor and inhale, lifting your arms, shoulders, and head, to come away from the floor as far as you can without straining (Fig. 17.85). Throughout this pose, keep your lower back toward the floor. Exhale and lower down slowly, coming back up on the next inhalation. Move in and out of this pose a few times before holding the upward position for 6 to 8 breaths. Exhale and lower back to the floor.

Bridge Pose (Setu Bandha Sarvangasana)

With your hands beside you, place your feet facing forward and as wide as they will go. Exhale and draw your lower back into the floor, your tailbone toward your pubic bone. Inhale and lift your hips as high as you can (Fig. 17.86). You can either stay on the floor with palms down or interlace the fingers, bringing the shoulder blades closer and drawing the hands down to the floor. If this wide stance strains your inner knees, turn the balls of your feet out more than the heels. Stay up for 6 to 8 breaths. Now, lying on your back with your knees bent and your feet resting on the floor, proceed to the next pose.

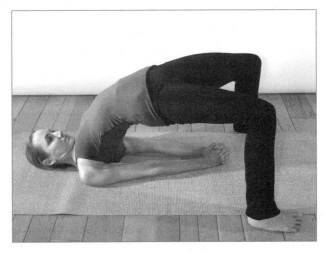

17.86. Bridge Pose (Setu Bandha Sarvangasana), Feet and Knees Wide Apart

Opposite Leg Abdominal Strengthener

Lying on your back, with your hands interlaced behind your head, bring your knees into your chest. Lift your left foot up with a straight leg. Exhale and draw your left elbow over toward your right knee as you extend out with your left leg (Fig. 17.87). Inhale and bring your body back to center, bend your left knee, straighten your right leg, and exhale over with your right elbow toward your left knee while extending through your right leg. Come back to center to complete 1 round. Try not to rest on whichever shoulder you are leaning toward; instead, bring your elbows closer together and center your weight. Continue moving side to side, breath by breath, for 5 rounds. Exhale and bring both feet to the floor as you rest your head back and release your hands to your sides.

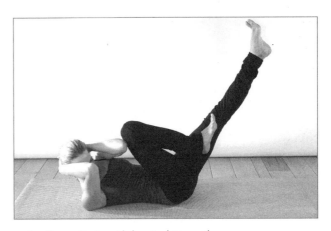

17.87. Opposite-Leg Abdominal Strengthener

Bridge Pose (Setu Bandha Sarvangasana)

Place your feet flat on the floor under your knees, hip-width apart. Exhale and draw your lower back toward the floor, keeping your hands beside you. Inhale and lift your hips as high as you comfortably can, drawing your tailbone toward your pubic bone and hugging your inner thighs toward each other, and keeping your hands on the floor near your hips (Fig. 17.88). Exhale and lower down vertebra by vertebra. Repeat this 6 to 8 times, and on the last lift, stay up for 6 to 8 breaths. Exhale and lower back down.

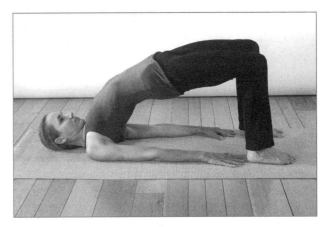

17.88. Bridge Pose (Setu Bandha Sarvangasana)

Lying Straddle Splits (Supta Konasana)

Bring your knees into your chest, then lift your legs straight up, spreading them as far apart as possible (Fig. 17.89). Place your hands on the inside of your knees, keeping your shoulders down, and exhale as you slowly bring your legs back together, using a little resistance with your hands (Fig. 17.90). On the next inhalation, spread your legs wide again, keeping your feet flexed. (Alternately you can place your feet on the floor against each other with the knees wide and continue with the same instructions; see Fig. 17.91) Repeat this 10 to 15 times.

On the last repetition, keep your legs wide and, on an inhalation lift your head and upper back and reach your hands between your legs with your fingers spread (Fig. 17.92). Stay in this position for 6 to 8 breaths. Exhale and lower your head and upper back to the floor. Rest your hands on your legs (Fig. 17.93), and stay in this position for 6 to 8 breaths. Exhale and bring your legs back together; bend your knees into your chest.

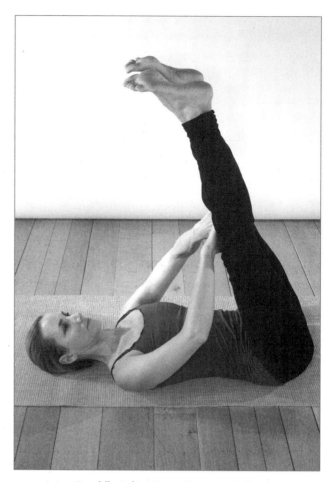

17.90. Lying Straddle Splits (Supta Konasana), Part 2

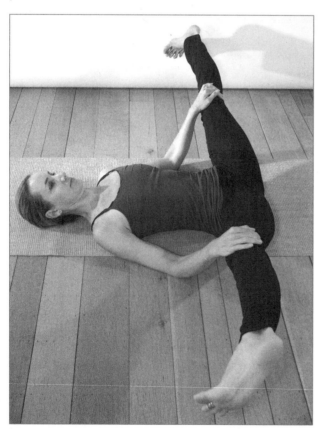

17.89. Lying Straddle Splits (Supta Konasana), Part 1

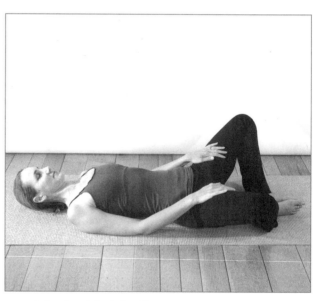

17.91. Lying Straddle Splits (Supta Konasana), Part 1 Variation

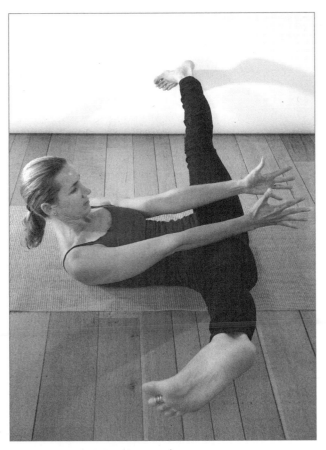

17.92. Lying Straddle Splits (Supta Konasana), Part 3

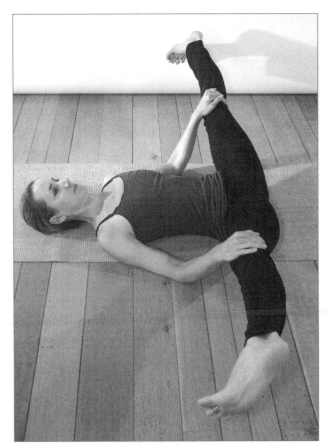

17.93. Lying Straddle Splits (Supta Konasana), Part 4

Knees-into-the-Chest Pose (Apanasana)

Rest in Knees-into-the-Chest Pose (Apanasana; Fig. 17.94), as described on page 100.

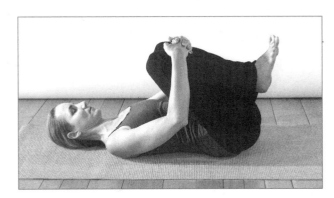

17.94. Knees-into-the-Chest Pose (Apanasana)

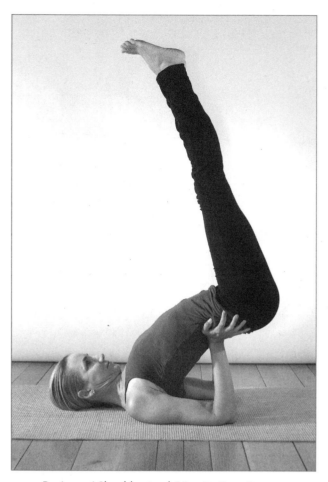

17.95. Beginners' Shoulderstand (Viparita Karani)

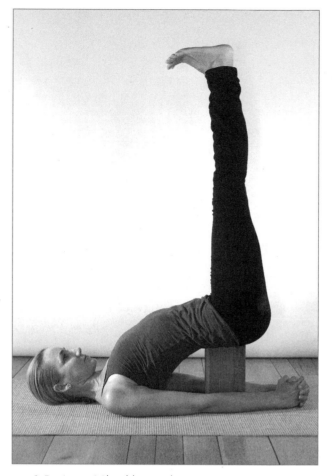

17.96. Beginners' Shoulderstand (Viparita Karani), Variation with Block

Inverted Action Pose or Beginners' Shoulderstand (Viparita Karani) with variations

If you are on the first three days of your menstrual cycle, have any neck injuries, or currently have an eye, ear, sinus, or tooth infection, or have high blood pressure, do not attempt any inversions such as this one. Rather, simply rest your back on the floor with your legs up the wall (Fig. 17.97).

From Knees-into-the-Chest Pose (Apanasana), lift your shins, tighten your abdominal muscles, and bring your knees near your head and, with your upper arms shoulder-width apart, place your hands under your lower back near your hips for support. Straighten your legs, reaching up through the balls of your feet (Fig. 17.95). Allow your upper back to move toward your chest, and press down with your upper arms. Keep your neck muscles unstrained, with a little lift in the back of your neck, resisting the temptation to tuck your chin into your chest.

If this feels like too much weight on your wrists, place a block under your sacrum and rest your arms at your sides, or clasped together (Fig. 17.96).

Stay in this pose for 10 to 20 breaths. Exhale and bend your knees toward your chest while using your abdominal muscles and hands, slowly rolling your back into the floor until the sacrum is down. With the knees bent, place your feet back on the floor and gently move your head from side to side. Then move your knees into your chest and interlace your fingers around your shins and rest for a few breaths.

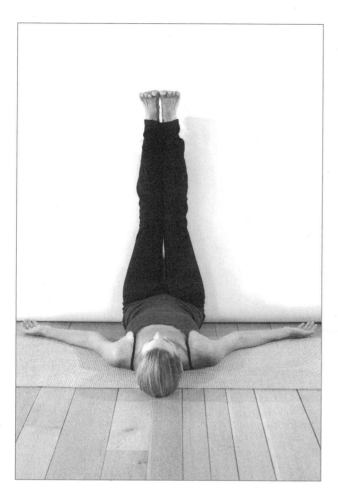

17.97. Legs-Up-the-Wall Pose (Viparita Karani)

Lying Spinal Twist Pose
(Jathara Parivatanasana)

Lying on your back with your arms out to the sides, inhale and bring both knees into your chest. Exhale and take your knees to the left while keeping the right side of your upper back on the floor. If your knees do not go all the way down, use a cushion to catch their weight. Bring your right arm up above the shoulder and rest it on the floor (or cushion). Turn your head to the right. Stay in this pose 1 to 3 minutes.

Exhale and lower your arm down by your side. Then inhale and, using your abdominals, bring your knees back to center before you exhale and drop them over to the other side, raising the left arm overhead and turning the head to the left. Stay 1 to 3 minutes. Exhale and lower the arm. Inhale and using your abdominals, bring your knees back into your chest (Fig. 17.99) (see page 123). Stay for 5 to 10 breaths.

Knees-into-the-Chest Pose (Apanasana)

Do Knees-into-the-Chest Pose (Apanasana) as described on page 100.

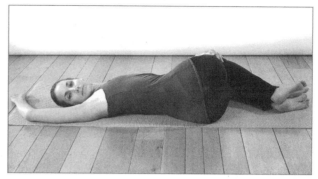

17.98. Lying Spinal Twist Pose (Jathara Parivatanasana)

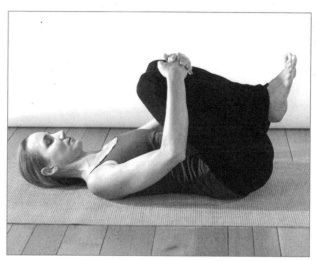

17.99 Knees-into-the-Chest Pose (Apanasana)

Corpse Pose (Savasana)

Do Corpse Pose (Savasana; Fig. 17.100) as described on page 47.

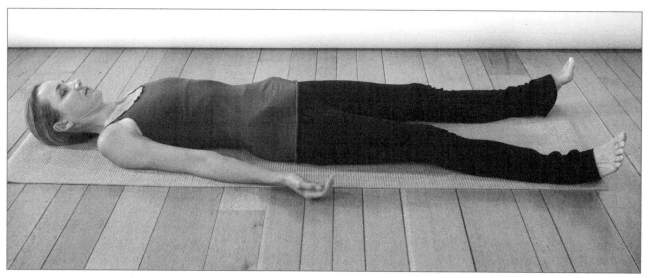

17.100. Corpse Pose (Savasana)

Fire-Building Yang Practice: Balancing the Lower and Upper Body

Sun Salutation
(Surya Namaskar)
with Lunges
(as shown on page 125)

 Standing Forward Bend (Uttanasana)

 Chair Pose (Utkatasana)

 Warrior I Pose (Virabhadrasana I)

 Chair Pose Part 2

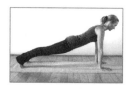 Plank Pose (Phalakasana)

 Mountain Pose

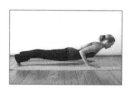 Four-Limbed Staff Pose (Chaturanga Dandasana)

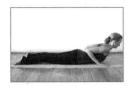 Cobra Pose (Bhujangasana)

Sun Salutation (Surya Namaskar) to Downward-Facing Dog Pose (Adho Mukha Svanasana) (same as above)

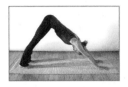 Downward-Facing Dog Pose (Adho Mukha Svanasana)

 Warrior I Pose (Virabhadrasana I)

Repeat Virabhadrasana I with right foot forward.

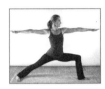 Warrior II Pose (Virabhadrasana II)

Sun Salutation (Surya Namaskar) to Downward-Facing Dog Pose (Adho Mukha Svanasana) (same as above)

 Extended Warrior Pose (Parsvakonasana)

 Warrior I Pose (Virabhadrasana I)

Sun Salutation (Surya Namaskar) to Downward-Facing Dog Pose (Adho Mukha Svanasana) (same as above)

Repeat the standing sequence with the right foot forward.

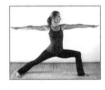 Warrior II Pose (Virabhadrasana II)

Sun Salutation (Surya Namaskar) to Downward-Facing Dog Pose (Adho Mukha Svanasana) (same as above)

Sun Salutation (Surya Namaskar) to Downward-Facing Dog Pose (Adho Mukha Svanasana) (same as above)

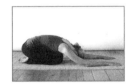 Child's Pose (Adho Mukha Virasana)

Repeat the standing sequence with the right foot forward.

 Dolphin Pose (Ardha Pincha Mayurasana)

Half-Handstand (Ardha Adho Mukha Vrksasana)

 Handstand (Adho Mukha Vrksasana)

 Headstand (Sirsasana)

Standing Forward Bend (Uttanasana)

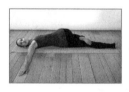 Lying Spinal Twist Pose (Jathara Parivatanasana)

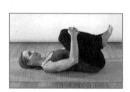 Knees-into-the-Chest Pose (Apanasana)

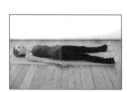 Corpse Pose (Savasana)

Sun Salutation (Surya Namaskar) with Lunges

Do the entire sequence (see page 125), with or without the lunge variations. Complete 1 to 5 rounds before proceeding to the next pose.

Chair Pose (Utkatasana)

From Mountain Pose (Tadasana), inhale and lift your arms overhead at shoulder-width. As you exhale, bend your knees into Chair Pose (Fig. 17.101). Inhale again, extending through your arms and hands. Exhale, bend your elbows and drop your head back (Fig. 17.102). Inhale as you straighten your arms up and look straight ahead, then exhale and draw your elbows down again with your head back. Repeat this for 6 to 8 breaths. Inhale and raise your arms, straightening your legs. Exhale and bring your hands in front of your heart in Mountain Pose (Tadasana) (Fig. 17.103).

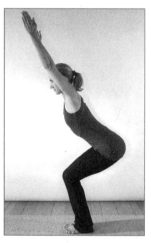

17.101. Chair Pose (Utkatasana), Part 1

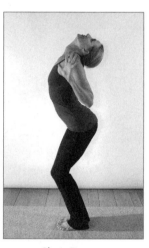

17.102. Chair Pose (Utkatasana), Part 2

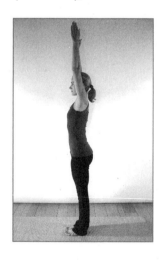

17.103 Mountain Pose (Tadasana)

Standing Forward Bend (Uttanasana)

From Mountain Pose (Tadasana), fold forward into Standing Forward Bend (Uttanasana; Fig. 17.104), as described on page 127. Stay in this pose about 1 minute.

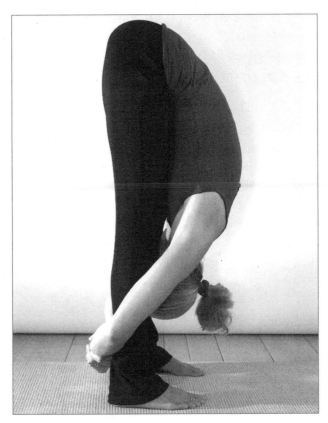

17.104. Standing Forward Bend (Uttanasana)

Warrior I Pose (Virabhadrasana I)

From the Standing Forward Bend (Uttanasana), inhale and lift the chest. Exhale and step one foot and then the other back to Plank Pose. Inhale in Plank, and then exhale to Four-Limbed Staff Pose (Chaturanga Dandasana). Inhale into Cobra, and exhale back to Downward-Facing Dog with the legs straight. Stay for 5 breaths. On the 6th inhale, step the left foot forward between the hands. As you exhale place the back edge of the right foot down with the toes facing more forward than the heel. Inhale and lift your torso with arms coming up above your head, shoulder width apart, and your hands facing each other (Fig. 17.105). Draw your right hip forward and your tailbone in. Lift up through the sides of your waist, your shoul-

ders, and your arms (keep your shoulders broad across your back by wrapping your outer underarms toward your chest. Track your left knee over your left foot, and deepen the lunge while pressing back through your inner right thigh and outer right foot. Keep the head centered and the gaze forward.

Stay in this pose 6–8 breaths.

To come out, exhale and bring your hands down and your back heel off the floor. Inhale and step back to plank, exhale to Four-Limbed Staff Pose (Chaturanga Dandasana). Inhale into Cobra, and exhale back to Downward-Facing Dog. Stay for 5 breaths. On the 6th inhale, step the right foot forward between the hands and repeat Warrior I on the other side.

To come out, repeat the sequence you did before (stepping back to Plank, Chaturanga Dandasana, Cobra, and so on) until you reach Downward-Facing Dog and stay there for 5 breaths.

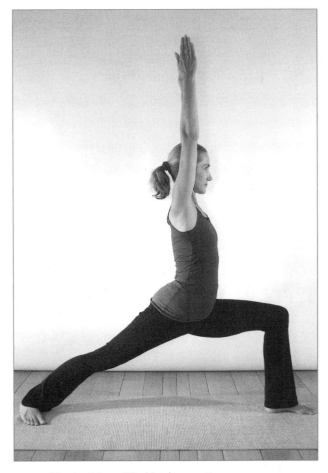

17.105. Warrior I Pose (Virabhadrasana I)

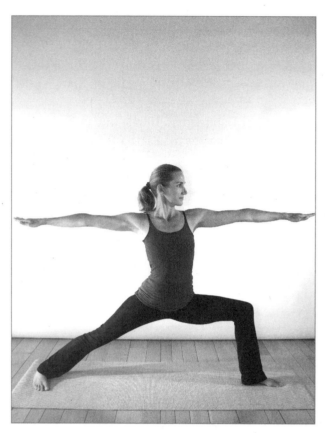
17.106. Warrior II Pose (Virabhadrasana II)

Warrior II Pose (Virabhadrasana II)

From Downward-Facing Dog, inhale and step the left foot forward (coming into Warrior I again, the same as before) for one breath. Take a breath in and as you exhale extend the front foot a little forward, open the hips to the side, and bring the arms down shoulder height, opening into Warrior II (Fig. 17.106). Allow your spine to be upright, centered between both legs, with your tailbone drawn slightly in and directed toward the left foot. Keeping the hips wide and your left knee centered over your left foot, hug your thighs toward each other while lifting your chest up and away from your waist, relaxing your shoulders down your back. Look out past your left fingers with a soft gaze. Stay in this pose for 6–8 breaths.

To come out, exhale your hands to the floor on either side of the left foot and lift off your back heel. Inhale as you step back to Plank Pose, exhale to Four-Limbed Staff Pose (Chaturanga Dandasana). Inhale into Cobra, and exhale back to Downward-Facing Dog. Stay for 5 breaths. On the 6th inhale, step the right foot forward between the hands and repeat Warrior I, opening into Warrior II on the right leg on the other side.

Come out of it the same way you did when your left foot was forward, exhaling the hands down and then inhaling in Plank, exhale to Chaturanga Dandasana, inhale in Cobra, exhale to Downward-Facing Dog for 5 breaths.

Extended Warrior Pose (Parsvakonasana)

From Downward-Facing Dog, inhale and step the left foot forward (coming into Warrior I again, same as before) for one breath. Take a breath in, and as you exhale, extend the front foot a little forward, open the hips to the side, and bring the arms down to shoulder height, opening into Warrior II again for one breath. Inhale, and as you exhale, extend your torso and left arm out to the side and down, bringing your right arm up and over your head past your ear with the palm facing down. Your left fingers can rest on the floor (Fig. 17.107) or a block near the outside of your left foot. Alternately, you can simply place your forearm on your left knee and allow your right arm to extend straight up above your right shoulder (Fig. 17.108). Keep your left knee drawn back above your left ankle while engaging your right inner thigh back toward your femur (thigh bone), resisting the pull toward the left lunge with the right leg. As you press your inner left foot down, draw your weight back into the outer edge of your right foot. Turn your ribs toward the sky, keeping your right underarm rotating toward the floor. You can alternate looking up under the arm toward the sky for a few breaths, with looking down at the floor a few breaths.

Stay in this pose 6–8 breaths.

Come out of it the same way you did before, exhaling the hands down on either side of the foot as you come off the back heel, and then inhaling in Plank, exhale to Chaturanga Dandasana, inhale in Cobra, exhale to Downward-Facing Dog for 5 breaths.

Repeat the above process (from Warrior I to Warrior II to Extended Warrior) with the right leg forward.

Come out of this series the same way you did before, exhaling the hands down on either side of the foot and then inhaling in Plank, exhale to Chaturanga Dandasana, inhale in Cobra, exhale to Downward-Facing Dog for 5 breaths.

Rest for 5 to 10 breaths in Child's Pose after you have completed the standing pose series above.

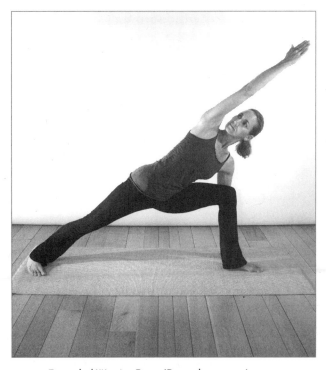

17.107. Extended Warrior Pose (Parsvakonasana)

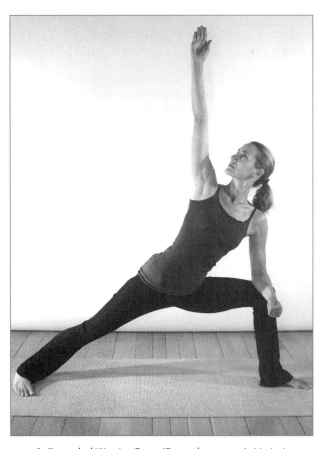

17.108. Extended Warrior Pose (Parsvakonasana), Variation

Dolphin Pose (Ardha Pincha Mayurasana)

From Child's Pose (Adho Mukha Virasana), raise your chest and place your elbows on the floor, shoulder-width apart, with your hands pressed together lightly. Inhale and lift off your knees, bringing your hips up and your chest back toward your legs (Fig. 17.109). Relax your head and continue to lift your shoulders away from your elbows and draw your torso toward your legs. Stay in this pose for 6 to 8 breaths. Exhale as you lower back to your knees.

Raise back up to Dolphin Pose (Ardha Pincha Mayurasana), then inhale and draw your right leg up, keeping your hips the same level. Straighten and extend up through your right leg while spreading your toes (Fig. 17.110). Maintain an even distribution of weight in shoulders, arms, and hands and continue to lift your weight away from your forearms. Stay in this pose for 3 to 6 breaths; lower your right leg as you exhale. Repeat the lift with your left leg. When you come down between sides, you can stay in Dolphin Pose or rest for a few breaths in Child's Pose.

Raise back up to Dolphin Pose (Ardha Pincha Mayurasana), but this time step your feet outside the width of your mat once your hips are raised (Fig. 17.111). Continue to lift away from your forearms and draw your weight back toward your legs for 6 to 8 breaths. Exhale as you come back down into Child's Pose (Adho Mukha Virasana).

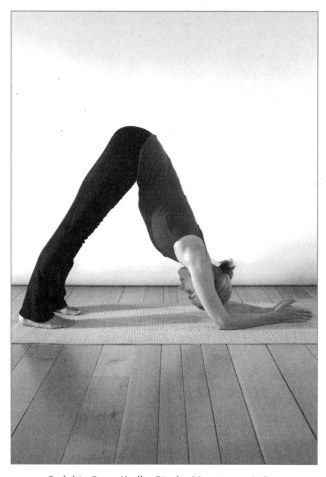

17.109. Dolphin Pose (Ardha Pincha Mayurasana), Part 1

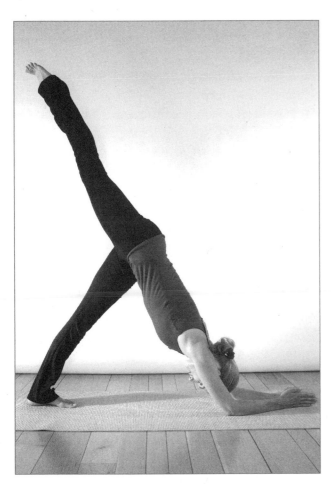

17.110. Dolphin Pose (Ardha Pincha Mayurasana), Part 2

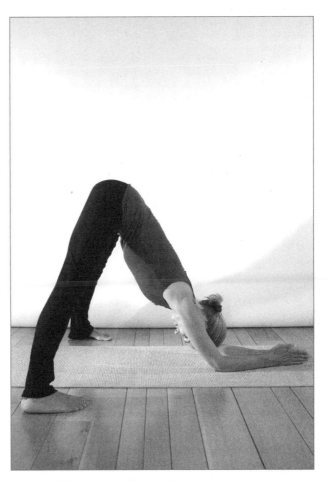

17.111. Dolphin Pose (Ardha Pincha Mayurasana), Part 3

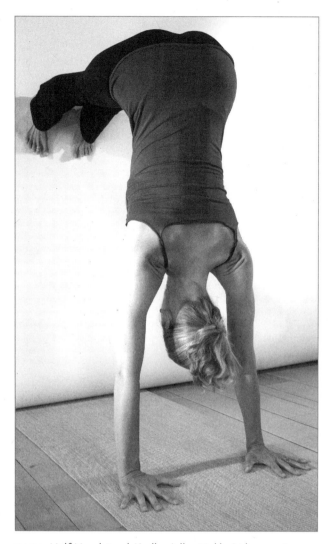

17.112. Half-Handstand (Ardha Adho Mukha Vrksasana)

Half-Handstand (Ardha Adho Mukha Vrksasana)

Take Downward-Facing Dog Pose (Adho Mukha Svanasana) with your heels resting on a wall. Then walk your hands a little closer to the wall. As you inhale, bring your right foot up to hip height against the wall with your knee bent; pause and exhale. As you inhale again, lift your left leg and place your left foot beside your right against the wall. As you exhale, slowly straighten your legs while bringing your chest toward the wall; keep your weight lifted away from your elbows and wrists, and your shoulders right above the wrists (Fig. 17.112). Relax your head and neck.

Stay in this pose for 8 to 10 breaths. Exhale and, bending the knees, step first the right foot down and then the left and rest for a few breaths in Child's Pose.

Handstand (Adho Mukha Vrksasana)

Note: This pose may require the assistance of a teacher for your first few times.

Place your fingers a hand's distance away from a wall and take Downward-Facing Dog Pose (Adho Mukha Svanasana). Walk your feet a foot closer to your hands, and inhale as you lift the right leg into the air. Keep the leg straight. Exhale and bend your left knee. Inhale and, with a lot of energy, lift your right leg up and then the left, straightening it right away and bringing both legs together until your feet touch the wall. Your weight will shift toward the wall as you kick up (Fig. 17.113). (If you are unable to reach the wall with both feet after several attempts, find a skilled yoga teacher to help you.) Once you are upright, engage your legs and spread your toes, lifting away from your hands and widening your shoulders. You can either look down at the floor (especially if you need help trying to balance), or relax the crown of your head toward the floor and use the wall for balance.

Stay in this pose for 6 to 8 breaths. To come down, keep one leg toward the wall and slowly bring the other one toward the floor on an exhalation, bending the knee as you land so it feels springy when

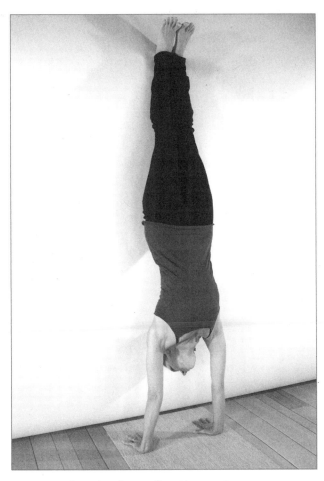

17.113. Handstand (Adho Mukha Vrksasana)

you make contact with the floor. Bring the other leg down, and rest in Child's Pose for a few breaths.

Headstand (Sirsasana)

Note: When we get to the stage of trying to balance in Headstand, I recommend you do so in the presence of a skilled teacher for your first few times.

From Child's Pose (Adho Mukha Virasana), bring your hands around your elbows to measure shoulder-width, then interlock your fingers with your forearms forward and your thumbs pointing up. Place the top of your head on a extra folded mat (near a wall if you are unsure of your balance), your weight just forward of your crown. Lift your knees and sitting bones as in Dolphin Pose (Ardha Pincha Mayurasana), and draw your torso toward your legs, keeping your shoulders away from your ears. Lengthen your underarms and draw your upper back in toward your chest. Come up on your toes, keeping your legs straight

and strong (part 1; Fig. 17.114). After a few weeks of this practice, try lifting one leg at a time up toward the sky for a few breaths, with your hips level and the rest of your body aligned as already suggested (part 2; Fig. 17.115). If this is too much on your hamstrings, bend your standing knee but keep your lifted leg straight.

Stay in each phase for 8 to 10 breaths before exhaling and lowering your leg, then inhaling and lifting the other leg. Rest in Child's Pose for a few breaths.

Even when you are able to balance in Headstand practicing parts 1 and 2 a few breaths before picking up can remind you how to align this pose properly.

To take a full Headstand (Sirsasana), it is best to practice it initially in the presence of a skilled teacher, as proper alignment is so important. If you already do this pose, simply place your arms and head as described before and bring one leg up toward the sky on an inhale; pause to exhale, use your abdominals, and distribute your weight equally through your arms. Inhale and lift your other leg, bringing your feet together overhead (Fig. 17.116). Remember to draw down through your forearms, up through your shoulders, in at your front ribs, up through your side, in at your tailbone, back through your thighs, and up through both feet. Keep scanning your body to realign your posture continually in this pose.

Stay in the pose 1 to 3 minutes. Come down on an exhalation, moving your feet forward and your hips back, using your abdominals as you pike your legs toward the floor. Keep your shoulders away from the floor the whole time you are coming

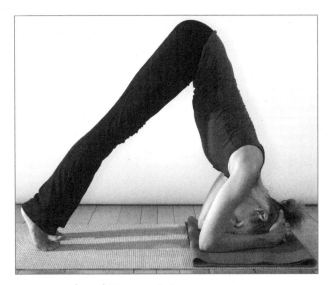

17.114. Headstand (Sirsasana), Part 1

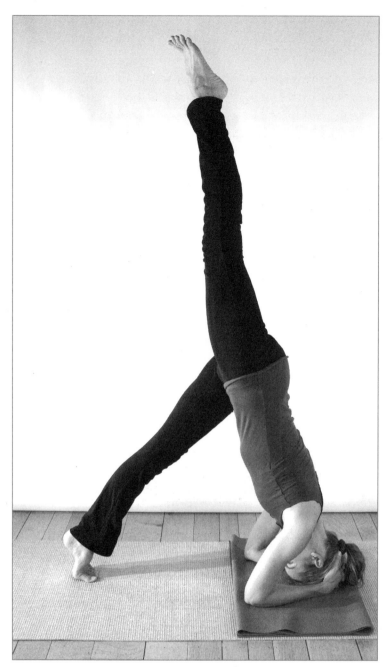

17.115. Headstand (Sirsasana), Part 2

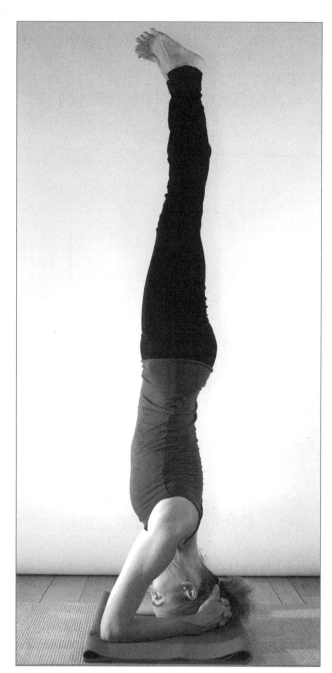

17.116. Headstand (Sirsasana), Part 3

down. Rest for at least 5 breaths in Child's Pose (Adho Mukha Virasana).

Standing Forward Bend (Uttanasana)

Do Standing Forward Bend (Uttanasana; Fig. 17.117), as described on page 127. Allow your hands to rest on the opposite elbows. Stay for one minute.

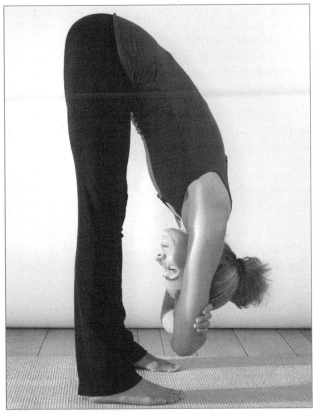

17.117. Standing Forward Bend (Uttanasana)

Lying Spinal Twist Pose (Jathara Parivatanasana)

Lie on your back and draw your right knee in toward you as you extend through the left leg. With the right arm placed out on the floor, exhale the right knee over to the left, keeping the right upper back on the floor. You can rest the left hand on the right knee while drawing the right hip away from the right ribs. Turn and look to the right. Stay for 10 breaths (Fig. 17.118).

To come out, exhale as you bring the right knee back over to the right and extend the leg. Bring the left knee in as you inhale and as you exhale, twist as before, this time with the left knee going over to the right and the left arm and upper back staying grounded to the left. Rest the right hand on the left thigh and draw the left hip away from the left ribs. Stay for 10 breaths.

Exhale as you release the twist and draw both knees into your chest, interlacing your fingers around your upper shins (Fig. 17.119).

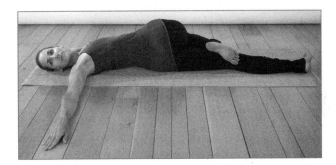

17.118. Lying Spinal Twist Pose (Jathara Parivatanasana) with One Leg Straight

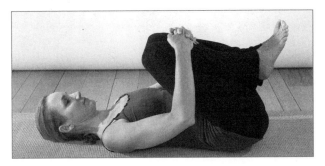

17.119. Knees-into-the-Chest Pose (Apanasana)

Knees-into-the-Chest Pose (Apanasana)

While lying on your back, bring both knees into your chest and interlace your fingers around your upper shins (Fig. 17.119). You can hold one end of a strap in each hand and loop this over your shins if you cannot bring your hands together.

Corpse Pose (Savasana)

Do Corpse Pose (Savasana; Fig. 17.122) as described on page 47.

After you have gone through your asana practices, it is essential to rest all your tissues in Corpse Pose (Savasana). This is an important time as your organism assimilates the added flow of chi and seeks a natural equilibrium. It is also a wonderful preliminary pose for meditation. You relax down into the floor and fully release all bodily holding. Psychologically, you let go of all effort and identification. You attempt to die as the person you have been in order to be born into a fresh innocence. If you truly practice this pose, you will simulate the dying process, letting go of everything you have been attached to, from your body to your loved ones, from your accomplishments and possessions to your history and plans. This complete release allows you to fully open to the mystery in front of you, the great unknown. As you relax deeply into the floor, closing your eyes, you are not preparing for a napping session, but instead are opening into a quiet alertness that is unhindered by any mental content or guidance. You cultivate a bright receptivity that lets go of all contrivance and self-reference, a freefall into the groundless ground. This full psychosomatic release of all tension, coupled with a clear alertness, becomes the foundation of your meditative awareness.

You should stay in this pose 5 to 15 minutes to allow a total release to occur in all layers of your being. If you find you have dropped off to sleep (which may happen often when you have been living your life in constant depletion), it is useful to do a brief pranayama practice to enliven the yang, alert side of your nature again before going into meditation.

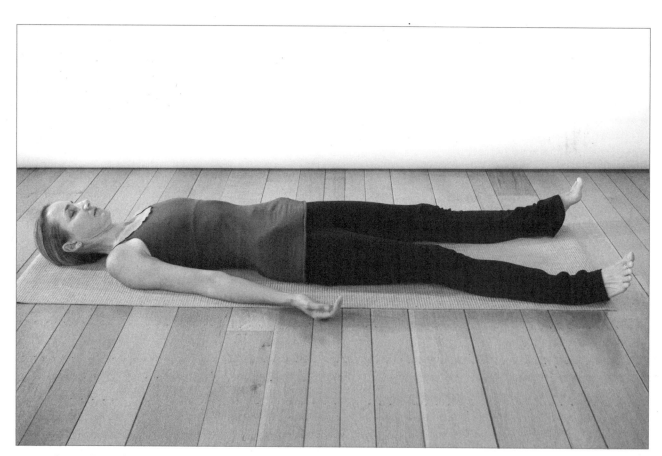

17.120. Corpse Pose (Savasana)

18

Seated Pranayama

PRANA MEANS "life force," and *yama* means "to enhance" or "to alter." Pranayama is a practice that enhances our pranic vitality and concentration skills by altering the three aspects of breathing; the inhalation (puraka), the exhalation (rechaka), and the pause in between (kumbhaka). It is a wonderful prelude to meditation because it calms and steadies the mind. It also helps clear blockages in the meridians, expels toxins from the blood, and rids the lungs of stale air. The rhythmic internal pressure stimulates the circulation of cerebral spinal fluid, bringing refined energy to the brain cells and glands, encouraging the center of the brain to work nearer to its optimal capacity, and the whole body is nourished by the extra supply of oxygen that is absorbed while carbon dioxide is efficiently expelled. Pranayama is especially recommended for people with insomnia, mental tension, or depression, and it is also said to help manage heart disease.

Generally, it is important to learn these practices in the presence of a qualified teacher, as we can disrupt our sensitive pranic system if we do not understand how to practice correctly. What I offer here is a simple yet effective collection of techniques that will help balance depleted resources of prana and bring a crisp alertness of mind, motivating us to begin a skillful seated meditation period. You can practice the short version of nine clearing cycles listed here either before or after your other practices. (I often do this practice before any asana or meditation practice.) When you have more time, you can practice one or more of the suggested styles after your asana practice and before your meditation.

Ida, Pingala, and Sushumna Nadis

Alternate Nostril Breathing activates and harmonizes the two main nadis that house our yin and yang energy, the ida and pingala nadis. Nadis are comparable to the meridians that conduct the flow of chi. Some say these two main channels correspond to the Urinary Bladder meridians on each side of the body. Others suggest the *du mai* channel is likened to the Pingala nadi (warm, solar, yang, energy) while the *ren mai* is similar to the concept of the Ida nadi (cool, lunar, yin energy). They are the seat of positive and negative charges in the body. We have already explored how our energy can be described in terms of its yin and yang qualities and how these labels change according to what we are comparing. If we look at the whole body and split it in half at the waist, the upper half would be considered yang and the bottom half yin. If we now take the body and dissect it through the middle from top to bottom, the energy that moves along the left side is considered yin in many traditions and the right side yang. Some lineages suggest that the opposite is true, and still others say the yin side is on the right in women, on the left in men, and the yang side is the opposite. For simplicity's sake, we will stay with the traditional Indian yogic description of yin on the left—considered the ida channel—and yang on the right—the pingala channel.

The origin and direction of these main channels are also described differently by different traditions. Some say they begin in the lower belly (svadisthana chakra) and crisscross up the spine like a helix, without touching each other or going directly through the other chakras (energy centers), until they join at the ajna chakra with the central channel (the sushumna), before separating again and ending in each nostril respectively. Others say the two main nadis begin in the base chakra, the muladhara, and run straight up either side of the central channel before joining at the third eye and coming down into the nostrils. Either way, these energetic twins circulate the receptive and radiant opposing energies that are connected with our dualistic mind states.

As we enter these channels consciously, distributing the chi exclusively along one corridor before enlivening the other, we begin to purify their energetic disturbances and bring them into a balanced, coessential harmony whereby the suspension of breath collects them into the center chakra (manipura). This begins to enliven not only the energy vortex at the center of our body (bridging the right and left, front and back, inner and outer energies), but the sushumna (central channel) begins to be enlivened as well, calling our attention inward toward our non-conceptual nature, our being beyond concepts. This energetic superhighway of the body passes through all the chakras along the center of the body, through the bone marrow, traveling to the crown of the head, and then dipping down to end in the area of the lower forehead, where it joins with the two side nadis, the ida and pingala, which end in the nostrils. (Note: some yogis declare that it does not flow along the in-

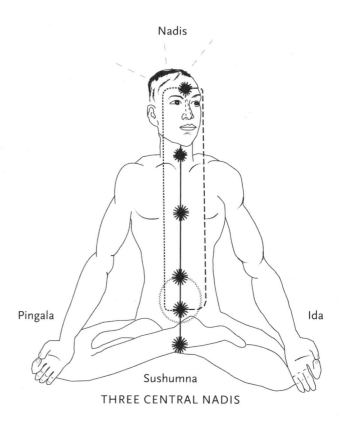

THREE CENTRAL NADIS

terior of the spine, but closer to the center of the body, in front of the spine.) The purpose of placing our attention in the two side channels is that when they are balanced, our consciousness begins to coalesce into the sushumna, the center of our body, allowing us to more easily segue into meditative awareness.

More advanced pranayama practices encourage dormant possibilities of inner expansion, often leading to deepened understanding of the most subtle realms of existence. To develop these skills, it is essential that you seek the mentorship of skillful guidance. If you or someone you know unwittingly wakes up regions of consciousness that cause antisocial, unskillful, bizarre, or risky behavior, you can look to the Spiritual Emergence Network (www.spiritualemergence.net) for referrals to therapists who are trained to discern the difference between authentic spiritual awakenings and neurotic or even psychotic disassociations and how to treat them appropriately.

Nine Clearing Cycles: A Seven-Minute Daily Breathing Practice

Sit in a comfortable, upright position, lengthening the vertical axis of your spine and placing your head back on top of your shoulders. Align your chin and forehead vertically. You can sit in any of the meditation postures suggested in chapter 20 (see page 179).

There is a simple hand position that easily allows us to alternate closing each nostril and keep a soft pressure point on the third eye. Do this by

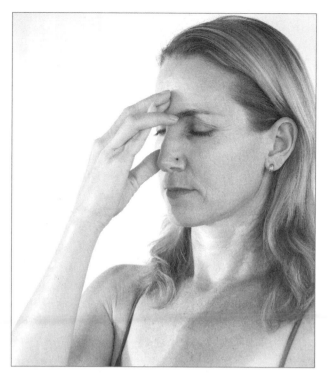

18.2. Breathing through the Left Nostril

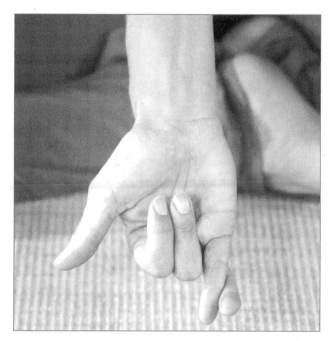

18.1. Hand Position for Alternate Nostril Breathing (Nadi Shodhana)

pressing together the first two fingers of your right hand and drawing your ring finger over to the outside of the little finger (Fig. 18.1).

To close your right nostril, press your thumb against the side of your right nostril and the tips of the first two fingers against your third eye (center of your forehead) (Fig. 18.2). Slowly inhale and exhale through your left nostril five times, allowing 5 seconds for each in breath, and about 5 seconds for each out breath. Then close the left nostril with the ring finger, lift the thumb, and take 5 slow breaths through the right nostril (Fig. 18.3). Now you begin the 9 clearing rounds. Close the right nostril with your thumb and through the left nostril allow a slow inhalation followed by a slow exhalation. Then breathe in slowly again followed by a brisk exhalation. These 4 breaths make up one round. Do three rounds. After three rounds on the left, close the left nostril, lift the thumb, and complete 3 rounds through the right nostril. Remember, the rhythm

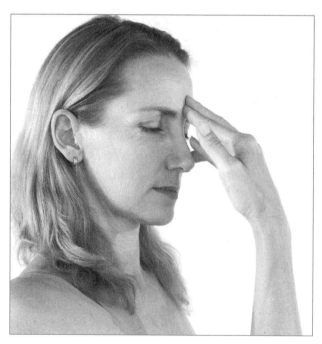

18.3. Breathing through the Right Nostril

of each round is in slow, out slow, in slow, out fast. After 3 rounds through both the right and left, bring your right hand down and do the same thing through both nostrils together for 3 rounds. This makes up 9 clearing cycles. (While you are exhaling on the left side, imagine you are letting go of your greed. While you are exhaling on the right side, you can aspire to release all your hatred. While breathing out through both nostrils, imagine releasing all your delusions.)

After the nine clearing rounds, inhale and hold the breath for about 10 seconds. Exhale very slowly and hold the breath again at the end of the exhalation for 5 to 10 seconds. Finish with three slow, full-body Ujjayi breaths.

This short but potent practice is good to begin the day, as it awakens the main energy center in your navel, which becomes more dormant during sleep and is the main energetic site from which we access our personal power.

Alternate Nostril Bellows Breath (Bhastrika)

Begin by closing the right nostril with your thumb, pressing your third eye with the first two fingers, and take five breaths in and out of the left side of your nose. While breathing in this way, guide your attention down the left channel to your pelvic floor on the in-breath and bring it back up the left side to your chest on the exhalation. Psychologically feel into the yin, contemplative, receptive side of your nature while breathing along the ida channel.

When you have taken five breaths, close your left nostril with your ring finger, open the right by lifting your thumb; repeat the same five breaths on the right. While breathing along this side, follow the right channel down on the inhalation and up on the exhalation, feeling into your yang, radiant, expressive side represented in the pingala nadi.

Repeat three times on each side.

Now take a breath in through your left nostril while closing the right, and rapidly breathe in and out for thirty "pumps" (or fewer if you lose the coordination along the way). If you falter, reduce it to ten rapid breaths in and out, pause and inhale, and then do ten more breaths. Complete three rounds through your left nostril. After thirty breaths on this side, close your left nostril with your ring finger, inhale through the right side of your nose, and repeat the same method, in and out rapidly for thirty pumps. When you have completed this, bring your right hand down and take

a slow Ujjayi breath through both nostrils. At the end of the inhalation, hold the breath for as long as feels appropriate for you (10 to 50 seconds is average in the beginning).

As you are holding the breath (kumbhaka), seal the prana into the center of your body by drawing your perineum in at the base of your pelvic floor (Root Lock [Mula Bandha]). During the suspension of breath, energy migrates more substantially to an area on which we concentrate. If during this pause in breathing, we create an inner vacuum by sealing the area with an internal physical action, we prevent prana from dissipating. This is called engaging a *bandha* (meaning "to bind or seal"). Bandhas not only redistribute and improve the flow of prana, but they also improve the health of the internal organs through the inner massage that occurs. They stimulate and regulate the nerves and remove stagnant blood, while releasing the energetic knots (*granthis*) that impede the flow of prana in the central region of the subtle body.

Root Lock (Mula Bandha) seals the lower portion of the energy pathways in our spinal column. To engage this bandha, we need to bring our attention to our pelvic floor. The perineum is located between the anus and the genitals and is a small, diamond-shaped muscle. This area acts as a chi bridge and redirects dissipating yin chi back up toward higher energy centers where it can join with the upper, or yang, chi. The perineum is the floor of the organs, and if it is allowed to become weak, energy leaks out. If our energy is redirected inward, we begin to feel grounded. To activate the perineum simply draw in your pelvic floor, as if you are trying not to go the bathroom. You may need to alternate pulling in with pushing down in order to bring awareness to this area. You can take a few breaths while you practice this. As you inhale, draw your attention down to the root. At the end of the inhalation, pause and lift your perineum up toward the center of your body (make this a lighter lift than squeezing the anal sphincter). Now let it drop and push down gently while you exhale. Mula Bandha is the act of subtly lifting the pelvic floor. Repeat this a few more times. Continue with the practice of pranayama with Root Lock (Mula Bandha).

Another place where energy easily leaks out is through the head. We can cap the energy off at the throat and seal it into the torso if we perform the Chin Lock (Jalandhara Bandha; *jal* means "throat" and *dhara* means "base"). It closes the trachea and compresses the nerves and glands of the throat, slowing the heartbeat, and sealing the top portion of the energy pathways in the spinal column. This bandha improves the function of the thyroid and parathyroid glands, which have a direct influence on our metabolism.

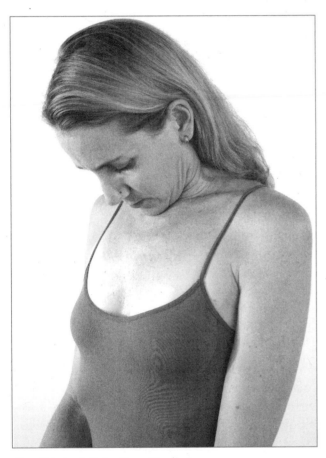

18.4. Chin Lock (Jalandhara Bandha)

To engage Chin Lock (Jalandhara Bandha), bring your chin forward and down to meet the top of your sternum with a soft pressure (Fig. 18.4). If you are unable to make physical contact, raise your shoulders slightly to lift your sternum and then bring your chin down to meet it.

When it is time to exhale, release the seals slowly and consciously so as not to force the breath out in one quick spurt. The bandhas cre-ate an internal pressure, like capping off a tube at both ends. When released, they create a geyser-like effect that pools chi into all the major meridians and acupuncture points, bathing your entire system in refined energy.

Repeat this process three times.

Alternate Nostril Breath with Kumbhaka

Having cleansed the two main channels, we will now inhabit each one separately, holding the energy in the center temporarily, and further encouraging the yin and yang (receptive and creative) energies to intermingle and join within us.

Begin by inhaling through your left nostril, closing the right with your thumb, and exhaling through the right, closing the left side with your ring finger. Then inhale through the right and exhale through the left. Allow each breath to last about 5 seconds as it comes in and about the same length of time as it goes out.

Repeat this for three rounds. On the fourth, inhale through your left nostril for 5 seconds, hold for 5 seconds, and exhale through the right for 5 seconds. Now begin an inhalation on the right side, hold for 5 seconds, and exhale through the left for 5 seconds. This is one full round. Repeat this for three rounds. Inhale left for 5 seconds, hold for 5 seconds, exhale right for 5 seconds— this is a ratio of 1:1:1.

Once you are able to repeat these three rounds without strain, you can add the bandhas. After a while, try and increase the kumbhaka (breath retention) to 10 seconds, allowing the exhalation to last 10 seconds also. Inhale left for 5 seconds, hold for 10 seconds, and exhale right for 10 seconds, a ratio of 1:2:2, then repeating on the other side for a ratio of 1:2:2.

Master Motoyama does not recommend increasing the ratios until you can complete twenty-five rounds comfortably. A good barometer in the beginning is to make sure you are able to exhale for the same amount of time that you just held the breath. So if you are breathing in for 5 seconds and holding for 10 to 15 seconds, you want to be able to exhale for 10 to 15 seconds as well. Eventually, as your energy body strengthens, you can increase the ratio to 1:4:2; in other words, inhale for 5 seconds, hold for 20 seconds, exhale for 10 seconds.

Once you are able to complete many rounds without straining, you can add a kumbhaka after the exhalation as well.

When holding the breath using the two bandhas already discussed (Mula and Jalandhara), you can also add a third one after the exhalation, the Belly Lock (Uddiyana Bandha; *uddiyana* means "flying back"). This bandha is a belly suction and further increases the pressure in the tube of the body to help pull stagnant chi up. It has a toning effect on the visceral organs, muscles, nerves, and glands by stimulating blood circulation and absorption. The heart is squeezed gently, creating an upward pressure that strengthens the diaphragm and all the respiratory muscles. This bandha also strengthens the digestion, elimination, and assimilation systems, while allowing for better absorption of oxygen and expulsion of carbon dioxide.

To create Belly Lock (Uddiyana Bandha), pause at the end of the exhalation. After you have completely emptied your lungs of air, lean forward a bit, and suction your abdominal cavity back under your ribs as much as you can (Fig. 18.5).

Using the bandhas together is called the Great Seal (Maha Bandha). This can be done with or without the fingers on the nostrils, but should be done only after exhaling. The three combined create an inner pressure in the center of our body. As we release, prana spreads throughout, toning, relaxing, and rejuvenating our entire system. These three locks together also help concentrate the upper and lower winds together into the core of the body. When these two energies meet at the navel, we naturally leave mundane concerns behind, cultivating more refined qualities of consciousness.

Usually, you will not be able to hold the breath out as long as you could hold it in. Try holding each one for only 5 seconds before allowing a slow, smooth inhalation. If you begin gasping for air after you have done this kumbhaka, hold it for less time on the following round.

The ratio for these rounds would be 1:2:2:1. Inhale left for 5 seconds, hold for 10 seconds, exhale right for 10 seconds, hold for 5 seconds. Then inhale right for 5 seconds, hold for 10 seconds, exhale left for 10 seconds, and hold for 5 seconds.

Repeat this for three rounds.

Skull Radiant or Breath of Fire (Kapalabhati)

Breath of Fire (Kapalabhati) is given so many accolades in the yogic texts that I want to list a number of them here to encourage you to practice this regularly. This rapid style of pranayama creates an internal rhythmic massage, stimulating the circulation of cerebral fluid and influencing the compression and decompression in the spine and brain. This stimulation pumps the diaphragm and lungs, improving the heart and blood circulation, which helps wash out waste gasses. It heats the nasal passages and sinuses, clearing away excess mucus, helping build up resistance to colds and respiratory disorders. It improves constipation and digestion, helps stimulate a sluggish system by accelerating the metabolic rate and strengthening the nervous system, and helps normalize the adrenals. This practice also accelerates pranic movement

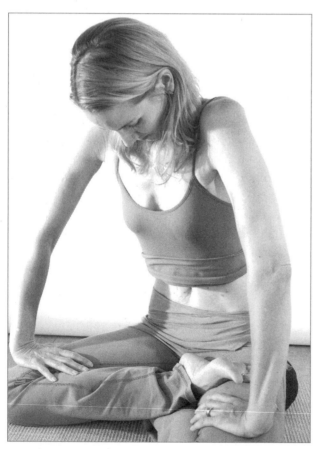

18.5. Belly Lock (Uddiyana Bandha)

throughout the body and brain, increasing physical vitality and bestowing clarity of mind.

You may want to begin by clearing your nasal passages by blowing your nose. Then choose a comfortable upright posture (see page 179 for suggestions). Begin by taking three slow Ujjayi breaths, placing one hand on your belly to stay connected to its movement. Take a full breath in and begin emphasizing the exhalation in quick, clear spurts similar to blowing your nose. Take short inhalations in order to keep going, but allow the emphasis to be on the exhalation. Do not close the front of your throat as you do in Ujjayi and do not push through your vocal chords. The sound is quick and crisp on the exhalation, silent on the inhalation. As you are pumping the exhalation out, remain steady in your posture, preventing your torso from swaying. Your spine will stay steady, while your belly moves in and out, matching the breath. Allow your hand to check your movements so that you feel the abdomen moving all the way back toward the spine as you exhale, relaxing briefly each time you inhale. The pace should feel consistent and repetitive.

Start with thirty pumps the first round, stopping sooner if you lose the rhythm of your belly moving in on the out-breath. On the last exhalation, slow the air a bit to allow all the breath out and then take a slow, deep Ujjayi inhalation and pause for a kumbhaka (breath retention) at the top of the inhalation.

Hold for 10 to 30 seconds using the Root Lock (Mula Bandha) and Chin Lock (Jalandhara Bandha) as explained previously. After holding the breath an appropriate amount of time (10 to 30 seconds), release the locks as you exhale, using Ujjayi in a slow and controlled manner. Take a full round of breaths when you have completed this. Repeat for three rounds.

With practice, you will strengthen your lungs and respiratory muscles, allowing you to easily increase the amount of pumps in each round. After a few weeks of consistent practice, you can allow one round to consist of fifty to a hundred pumps. A good way to count the number of breaths as you go is to put your hands in a soft fist on your thigh. Each time you complete ten pumps, let one finger come out. This method gives you a way to keep track of the appropriate number for you, as it will

vary from person to person and week to week. Stay with however many pumps you can comfortably do for at least a few weeks before extending it.

Kumbhaka

In the section on Alternate Nostril Breathing (Nadi Shodhana), we saw how this practice can improve the oxygen supply in the blood as well as direct more concentrated amounts of chi into any area we focus on. This practice can be included after the other styles, or it can be practiced on its own.

Sitting in an upright posture, take three deep Ujjayi breaths, focusing your mind into the central channel (sushumna). Take about 5 seconds to complete the next inhalation, and when you are full, hold the breath for 10 seconds. During the suspension of breath, engage the Root Lock (Mula Bandha) and Chin Lock (Jalandhara Bandha), while resting your concentration at the navel region, where the yin and yang energies join.

Hold for 10 to 50 seconds, depending on your capacity. *Do not strain.* As you begin the exhalation, release the locks and allow your out-breath to be slow and even, taking about 10 seconds to complete it. If this causes any strain or the exhalation is much shorter than the length of time you held the breath, then shorten the kumbhaka.

The ratio here is 1:2:2. Repeat this for three rounds.

After a few months of this practice, you can add three rounds of holding the breath after exhalation. It is not as easy to hold the breath after exhalation as it is after inhalation, so start with a length of time that is not stressful for you. Begin with 5 seconds on the inhalation, exhaling for 10, and holding the breath for 5 after you exhale. As you engage the kumbhaka, include the Root Lock (Mula Bandha) and Chin Lock (Jalandhara Bandha) as well as the Belly Lock (Uddiyana Bandha). Make sure you are empty of air before suctioning your belly back and holding the breath.

The ratio here is 1:2:1. Repeat this for three rounds.

Great Seal (Maha Bandha)

After a few months of practicing the pranayama I've just described, you can try three rounds of holding after each breath. Make sure you do not strain in any way and that the breath following the kumbhaka is as long as the time you held it. You can engage Root Lock (Mula Bandha) and Chin Lock (Jalandhara Bandha) after the inhalation and add Belly Lock (Uddiyana Bandha) when you are holding after the exhalation performing Maha Bandha, the Great Seal.

Inhale for 5 seconds, hold for 10, then exhale for 10, and hold for 5. The ratio here is 1:2:2:1. Repeat for three rounds.

19

Basic Buddha-Dharma

MINDFULNESS TRAINING stems from the teachings of the Buddha, given more than twenty-five hundred years ago and codified as one of the limbs of the famous Noble Eightfold Path. Mindfulness is both an attitude and a technique that is encapsulated within the practice of *vipassana* (insight). *Passana* means "to see" or "to recognize," and *vi* means "a special way." So vipassana is the art of seeing or relating to life freed from the mesmerizing power of our entrenched prejudices and preferences. This unconstricted view breeds insight into the underlying nature of things. Mindfulness is the practice that develops this kind of seeing. In order to practice mindfulness well, it is helpful to be acquainted with the fundamental principles of this path.

The Buddha's profoundly inclusive but radical perspective begins with contemplating the meaning of true well-being. He pointed out the ubiquitous desire to experience happiness is a common and universal motivation in all people. How we define happiness and what attitudes and behaviors arise in our pursuit of it ultimately determine the quality of our lives.

The Buddha then described eight conventional attitudes that dominate our mind states, providing the fuel for our unskillful fantasies and behaviors. He called these polarized dichotomies the eight worldly dharmas, which are four pairs of opposite themes:

What We Want	What We Don't Want
Pleasure	Pain
Praise	Blame
Recognition	Disgrace
Gain	Loss

Most of us unwittingly find ourselves in the insidious snare of this formula, duplicitously swinging between an irrepressible attempt to manifest and hold on to the first list and a furtive compulsion to avoid the second list. This, we assume, is the recipe for happiness. The inherent problem with this uninvestigated template is that it instills a primordial tension between what we crave and what we dread. It locks us into a furious insistence that conditions must conform to our desires in order for us to be happy, and of course, conditions arise autonomously, without consulting us. The only consistency we can count on is the inevitability that things will change. So no matter what we achieve or acquire, our hearts will eventually break when conditions shift.

The Buddha's simple and profound experiential insight is that the second list, involving pain, blame, disgrace, and loss is inevitable, as well as sickness, old age, and death. He suggested that we learn to contemplate these features of life as truly unavoidable and universal rather than as proof of our humiliating inferiority or punishment from some diabolical power. He also suggested that before we try to change conditions, we should learn to investigate our relationship to whatever is happening in us or to us (rather than oppressively suffocating in the entrapment of each uncontrollable event), assuming that life has somehow betrayed some secret promise to us. While initiating change is often appropriate, denying or wrestling with adverse circumstances while trying to hold on to the comforts of pleasure and praise will never allow us to rest in true contentment.

The Buddha claimed that there is a less precarious form of happiness available to anyone willing to take up a path of inquiry. His teachings suggest that the root of authentic happiness stems from living in such a way that our hearts and minds expand to include all eight worldly dharmas. Although it sounds impossible at first, we can actually learn to live inside pleasure *and* pain, gain *and* loss. Instead of trying to get rid of or deny difficult experiences, we learn to open to these intrinsic vulnerabilities without cutting off from the direct experience of them. Through meditative attention, we investigate for ourselves the liberating possibility of ending the struggle with pain, blame, disgrace, and loss.

Sincere mindfulness practice can only arise out of a deep interest in probing these inescapable features in our existence. We have to be curious about how we might sensitively learn to relate to all of life's experiences in more conscious ways. The Buddha's teachings and practices breed insight into a deeper meaning of happiness by teaching us how to connect nondefensively with life's ephemeral conditions, laying the groundwork for ever-more subtle levels of inquiry about the deeper nature of being.

The Three Jewels

If we are interested in relinquishing the struggle with existence, we must begin to recognize all the ways we are attached to promoting pleasant circumstances and at war with the unpleasant. For this complex endeavor, we need some strong support. The Buddha's path offers us this assistance in the form of a threefold system called the three jewels, which are the Buddha, the dharma, and the sangha. The Buddha in this context is our awakened nature (reflected in the historical teacher we call the Buddha). Under our patterns of conditioning lies our buddha-nature, or what could also be called open awareness, our true inner home. As we train in maintaining meditative attention with various features within our experience, over time we learn to rest in the spacious field of attention itself. Whatever the content of our experience, our sense of security or refuge becomes the unfettered, borderless realm of awareness itself.

The dharma of the three jewels refers to all of the Buddha's teachings on the nature of reality. We need to contemplate and practice these teachings in order to recognize and stabilize our ground of being. These tools keep us on the authentic path of awareness; they are the roads home.

The sangha is the community of people who are on this investigative path, who live in or aspire to live in awareness. They are our teachers, mentors, and friends who encourage us along the way and help us regain our footing when we falter. They are our spiritual family.

The three jewels become precious to us as invaluable support, our refuge throughout life. Rather than wandering in the cyclical habits of our unconscious patterns, or *samsara* (which literally means "to go round and round"), taking refuge in the three jewels leads us home to our full potential for psychological freedom. This kind of happiness manifests as a dynamic and direct relationship with the mystery of life, a life motivated by a passionate desire to live free of the entrapments of greed, hatred, and delusion. This is called nirvana.

> Whether or not buddhas appear, the truth remains the same. Heaven and hell are not topographies, but exist as states within our own minds.
>
> —*Buddha*

The Four Noble Truths

Over thousands of years, the Buddhist path has morphed into varying styles of behavior and practice, yet the common denominator among all schools is the primacy of the four noble truths. These simple but profound themes are not simply concepts in which we need to believe, nor did the Buddha invent them. He merely arranged these essential subjects together, emphasizing often overlooked insights into the nature of suffering and the possibility of its release. These four truths are interdependent and must be understood collectively if we are to progress along the path. If we isolate the first noble truth from the others and fail to hear the whole story, we may misinterpret the Buddhist path as depressing rather than practical and optimistic.

The first noble truth states that life has suffering. Suffering manifests for all of us in myriad ways, including stress, fear, tension, anxiety, depression, disappointment, abandonment, estrangement, anger, terror, jealousy, shame, and so on. Even if we have been graced with a wonderful life, take impeccable care of our bodies, have healthy genes and a strong constitution, we will eventually get sick, grow old, and die. No riches, surgery, drugs, or vaccinations can protect us from this indisputable truth. Learning to graciously accept life's inherent difficulties decreases our tendency to feel betrayed by circumstances. This frees us to relate to things more honestly and directly.

In each truth, there is an implied injunction to respond to life in a profoundly inquisitive and direct way. The imperative in the first truth is to investigate all the ways we suffer. We learn to turn our attention toward every aspect of ourselves without censorship. This kind of unbiased attention breeds insight into the changing nature of existence (anicca), the distinctive feature of Buddhist meditation. As we contemplate all the ways we feel disturbed while simply sitting still, we begin to have glimpses of the underlying fluidity of each sensation, emotion, and thought. Even when we suffer, we eventually begin to experience the lack of solidity in whatever we are struggling against. During this process, we learn to suffer consciously and authentically, paving the way for reducing and eventually relinquishing our suffering.

The first truth lays out the situation in which we find ourselves, and the second points to its cause. The second noble truth states that we suffer because of our grasping habits, which stem from ignorance about our deeper being. Here, the Buddha reduces all of our struggles to the all-pervasive attitude of grasping, which refers to all the ways we hold on. Clinging, as grasping is also called, is so insidiously ingrained and prevalent that it often remains hidden from our consciousness. Our sophisticated denial mechanisms can easily obscure this root of all afflictions. The injunction here is to relinquish our grasping, first in small ways and eventually moving on to our more entrenched tendencies.

The third noble truth refers to the possibility that we can cease grasping, leading to the extinction of suffering. Remember that pain is inevitable and suffering, being a state of mind, is optional. Here is the optimistic news that can motivate us along the path. The Buddha was confident in the underlying capacity of sincere aspirants to find true freedom. With himself as the example, he encouraged us to persevere in the face of all seemingly impervious obstacles, inspiring us to realize our unbounded nature as the fruition of this path. The action in the third truth is realization.

The fourth noble truth gives us the tools to experience true happiness or freedom from suffering and comprises the noble eightfold path. It is considered noble because our true inheritance is not based on birth or rank, but on the quality of our understanding about our fundamental nature. When these truths are integrated into the depth of our being, they are considered ennobling, elevating our character to the height of royal dignity. The action at this phase is one of continuous cultivation.

The Three Cardinal Points

The eight limbs of the eightfold path are composed of teachings and practices to directly influence our being and behavior. These include wise view, wise thought, wise speech, wise action, wise livelihood, wise effort, wise mindfulness, and wise concentration. All eight aspects are considered essential, yet three are given particular importance because without them, none of the other principles can take root in us. They are wise view, wise effort, and wise mindfulness, and they are called the three cardinal points. Many wonderful resources about the eightfold path are available, and I have listed some in the Selected Readings section at the back of this book. For our present purposes, I will focus on view, effort, and mindfulness.

Wise View

The first of these points to the overarching importance of our worldview. The Buddha listed two essential aspects needed for us to have an intelligent outlook on life:

- An understanding of cause and effect
- A deep understanding of the four noble truths

The first aspect of this teaching is contemplating the relationship between action and reaction, cause and effect. Every situation is preceded by a number of elements coming together to make that situation arise, what could be defined as a confluence of interdependent aspects creating a consequence. For example, a full-grown tree is an effect of many coessential elements that collide as initial causes. A seed blown by the wind is eventually wrapped in nourishing soil, sun, and rain, causing the effect of growth in specific patterns. Similarly, suffering can be thought of as an effect that arises out of a number of causes. Learning to examine the roots or causes of suffering and

diminish and eventually extinguish them is the essence of the Buddhist path.

Inquiry is one of the fundamental means to breed insight into suffering. We cultivate an excavator's curiosity about the conditions needed for us to become embedded in suffering. Although we may not overtly cause the problems we face, our attitude toward what happens is what we become interested in and is ultimately the deciding factor that determines whether we suffer or not. For example, if we know that every time someone suggests an alteration to our behavior we react with isolating rigidity, we can—through our mindfulness practice—investigate, loosen, and see through defensiveness (the cause of our tension). Now we have a choice about how we respond rather than compulsively giving in to an inevitable knee-jerk reaction. We may still feel the trigger as an inner constriction initially, but we no longer feel blindly compelled to act out from this inner event. We now have mindfulness tools that allow us to directly connect with what is going on inside. Since we are investigating our experience instead of fully identifying with it, the charade of invincibility is not given our full allegiance this time, inevitably creating a different effect under the same circumstances that caused us to suffer before.

The second aspect of wise view involves contemplating the four noble truths. The Buddha called suffering an all-pervasive dissatisfaction, a sickness, and comprehending the four noble truths was the cure. As is commonly suggested, we can look at these truths from a medicinal point of view. Like a doctor, the Buddha confirmed that we are sick and suffering—the first noble truth. In the second truth, he diagnosed the cause of this illness as our fixated grasping. In the third, he affirmed our capacity for a full recovery, freedom from suffering, which will manifest as wisdom and compassion. In the final truth, he prescribed the remedy that can cure us, the noble eightfold path. Like any patient, if we have seen a trusted doctor but do not actually take the prescribed medicine, we will not get well. To arouse a wise view, we must take up the eightfold path so we can fully understand and relinquish suffering and then realize and cultivate the path to freedom from suffering.

Wise Effort

Wise effort is the second cardinal point. This teaching reminds me how crucial it is that we have a storehouse of energy to draw from when studying ourselves and that we learn how to use it well. The Buddha reminded us that we need to use diligent and sustained effort to overcome the momentum of habitual patterns of reactivity and disconnection. We are counseled to make an effort to abandon unwholesome mind states and to cultivate wholesome ones. Unwholesome mind states are called the five hindrances; they are the compulsive thoughts and feelings that inevitably oppress us. These five universal afflictions chronically arise in each of us, often masquerading as appropriate responses to seemingly untenable circumstances. At times they will be obvious, while at other times they can linger in the shadows of our awareness, remaining devilishly subtle and cloaked in indignant self-righteousness. When we relate to these patterns nondefensively, they become workable and often beckon us toward greater self-discovery. The five hindrances are craving, aversion, restlessness, lethargy, and doubt.

Chasing after sensual gratification is the main ingredient in craving. It occurs when we are seduced by pleasant memories, fantasies, or experiences and fixate on holding on to or creating more of them. This attitude has a hypnotic and intoxicating quality that can easily remain hidden from our intelligence and awareness, even as it takes us under.

Aversion is when we resist, resent, recoil, attack, or become annoyed or impatient; in other words, when we reject any aspect in ourselves or our experience because we are unable to tolerate the unpleasantness of how we feel. This hindrance severs our ability to investigate ourselves more closely, since it is psychologically impossible to authentically examine something that we are resisting. These first two mind states (craving and aversion) are what fuel our struggle with existence and are the main expressions of our suffering.

Restlessness and mental lethargy are twins of a similar sort to craving and aversion and manifest as habitual coping strategies that stem from an underlying discontent. Like channel surfing with the television remote, when we are neither stimulated nor interested in the content of a moment, our mind can swing between two insatiable extremes: we either recklessly jump about from one detail to another, anxiously searching for something to cling to, or we simply sink into a hazy, vague disconnect and spaciness, neither of which brings sincere satisfaction. Lethargy and restlessness are often superficial symptoms that stem from deeper feelings of historical discontent and disappointment that ferment in the shadows, motivating unskillful behaviors such as boredom and mental laziness. (Note that this is different than true physical exhaustion and can only be properly diagnosed when we have gotten the deep rest of which we often deprive ourselves and still find our consciousness sinking.)

Doubt is a category all on its own because it stems from a myriad of entrained thought patterns embedded in our self-image. This hindrance can be the most paralyzing of all, as it freezes us in a construct of unrelenting self-talk that has already convicted and sentenced us to defensiveness. Doubt here is much different than inquiry or not knowing; it leaves no room for possibility, assuming conclusions without sincere investigation. This hindrance grows out of an overriding but hidden agenda to avoid our innermost fears and tragically keeps us from seeking out the help we need to break free from the shackles that bind us.

These five afflictions and their many variations become overwhelmingly apparent for each of us as we become intimate with our inner world through sitting practice. Knowing this, we can begin to recognize these patterns as universal demons of our conditioning with no substantial or inherent existence on their own. Through the process of exposing these fixations to nonjudgmental, nonreactive attention, we begin to recognize their cunningness sooner, learning to distrust their malicious provocations. What is required is a willingness to accept and interact with all the inner anguish we find inside us. This renders each emotion more permeable and less threatening, as they are no longer split off from the light of our compassionate attention and awareness. The afflicted state literally becomes permeated with caring attention, causing it to shift into something else that is often more tender and vulnerable. Each affliction we turn toward becomes a sacred doorway into greater emotional intelligence and capacity.

Although working with our obstacles is one of the most challenging aspects to this practice (and often why neophytes abandon ship), it is also the most profoundly liberating aspect that arises out of a mindfulness practice. The hindrances do not actually go away as a result of practice; we simply stop fighting with or ignoring them. Since we no longer feed them our abiding allegiance, they become starved into extinction. This is called momentary liberation. We are not magically relieved of all future reactivity, but everything begins to taste differently as we change our diet. Like breath, they come in, are given our nonjudgmental attention, and eventually flow out of us with less and less ability to cause capricious catastrophes.

A common instruction for acknowledging the presence of a hindrance is to name its appearance. As we sit and watch our breath, we might find ourselves drifting off into a pleasant fantasy; in coming awake to this diversion, we silently note that this is craving and simply return to our breath. When I was training in vipassana on my first ten-day retreat with S. N. Goenka, I found myself struggling painfully to follow the most simple meditation instructions each day. I watched my torturously restless mind bolt off every other moment, while my body's aches and pains felt punishingly unrelenting.

Each predawn morning, I summoned my inner warrior to help me endure another agonizing day of arduous stimulus deprivation, determined to stay the course and not collapse into the inner anguish I was feeling. By the end of each day, it took everything I had not to break down, admit defeat, and bolt out of there. On about the fourth day, I started settling down enough to actually hear some of the instructions meant to support the long hours in meditation. Goenka's thick Indian accent began to soothe and comfort me as his voice would break through the restless silence of shifting, coughing, and sighing meditators

and invite us to "watch our desperation." I was so relieved to hear him acknowledge and name my seemingly isolated and pathetic experience, and my relentless self-pity abated somewhat.

By day six, I knew I could make it the whole ten days, happily surprised to be able to tap into unexpected pockets of true serenity and insight. It wasn't until that afternoon that I was mentally clear enough to hear what Goenka's instruction had actually been all along. He had not been asking us to note our "desperation"; he had simply been suggesting that we "watch our *respiration*." Laughter jumped out of me into the silent space as I realized my projection of emotional support had been in my mind all along, just as the desperation had been.

I left the retreat with the inspiring realization that meditation could carve open all the fissures of my mind and expose the many delusions stored inside, helping me to see what lay beyond them. This, I decided, would be a worthwhile lifelong endeavor. I also decided that if I were to teach meditation to others one day, I would remember to acknowledge the realm of desperation, helping people to open to all their emotions and to relate to them as precious doorways into the strength of vulnerability.

Wise Mindfulness

The third cardinal point is wise mindfulness. In stressing the importance of mindfulness, the Buddha emphasized the necessity of meticulously examining the body and mind. This practice brings us into a direct relationship with the roots of suffering (our patterns of reactivity) and ultimately stimulates insight into our deeper wisdom nature. As we begin to understand ourselves better, we relax our compulsions to react out of habit.

This meticulous inquiry into the nature of existence trains us to discriminate between awareness and the objects of awareness. We learn to recognize the distinction between that which is constantly changing—for example, the breath—and that which is constantly available, such as the awareness that knows the breath. This discernment diminishes our tendency to grasp at the ungraspable (those features that are in constant flux).

The Buddha helpfully pointed out that everything that exists, from a mountain lake to a crying baby, is inextricably dependent on various causes and can therefore be called conditioned. He taught that everything conditioned is composed of three characteristics worthy of our contemplation and personal investigation. Ignorance of these three truths is the motivation for grasping and the root cause of suffering. These three characteristics are impermanence (anicca), unsatisfactoriness (dukkha), and selflessness (anatta).

The common denominator among all manifest existence is the birth and death process. Everything manifest was at some point nonexistent; arose out of certain conditions coalescing; changes during its life cycle; and eventually, as features shift and destabilize, deteriorates and expires. This organic cycle of constant metamorphosis is the meaning of impermanence. Investigating impermanence on all levels of our being is the fundamental theme of Buddhist meditation. Mindfulness can be described as an awareness of change. Understanding the precious impermanence of each seemingly ordinary moment fosters an unconstructed immediacy and intimacy with life.

The second characteristic is the intrinsic unreliability of impermanent existence. Since change is a constant, we cannot count on anything staying the same indefinitely. Ignorance of this fact causes us to compulsively consider permanent that which is inherently ephemeral. We naturally hold on to whatever we cherish, feeling betrayed when we lose these objects of attachment. Whatever we cling to unconsciously will cause us to suffer from its loss. Struggling with this seemingly cruel inevitability of change causes anguish, or dukkha. *Dukkha* is also translated as "anguish" or "suffering." Things and people are not ultimately unsatisfying because of their impermanent nature, but because we cling to the idea of their permanence.

The third characteristic recognizes the interdependency of all things. The Buddha suggested that we contemplate how nothing in the manifest universe exists in isolation as an independent entity. He described reality as a confluence of interdependent coarisings, empty of permanence. This lack of an independent self-nature is called selflessness, or anatta. Although we think of a tree as a separate solid entity, if we remove the wood, the soil, the sun, and the air, we have no tree. It is empty of an eternal, independent tree self. In the same way, our sense of "I" seems isolated, yet like the interdependent parts of a tree, we are a collection of aggregates that make up a temporary, self-organizing center, inseparable from and vulnerable to changing characteristics. Investigating the cherished assumption of a solid self is the main motivation for Buddhist meditation practice. Mindfulness leads to a discovery of the natural realm of vast awareness, refreshingly replacing the need to grasp at a permanent self.

The Four Foundations of Mindfulness

Training in mindfulness involves four interrelated domains of experience called the four foundations of mindfulness. These four spheres of introspection include the body, feelings, mental formations, and objects of mind.

The First Foundation of Mindfulness

Learning to clearly examine each pleasant and unpleasant aspect of our experience without prejudice begins to breed insight into the inherent lack of solidity in each seemingly independent feature. We begin to see for ourselves that when we look closely at any element of our experience, it disperses into many distinct and porous features, each of which can become a new object of our attention. Our back pain, for example, becomes a kaleidoscope of shooting, heavy waves that come and go from breath to breath, and each wave has a different intensity, length, and location. Each location pulsates differently, feeling like empty space one minute and sharp rays of intensity the next. This is the first foundation of mindfulness—mindfulness of the body. While being mindful of the body, we do not try to prevent or ignore pain (or pleasure, as the case may be). Instead, we have the direct, unmitigated experience of the sensory world unfolding within us. We attempt to relax into a participatory observation of all of our sensations, whether they are deliciously pleasant, maliciously unpleasant, or neutral and banal.

The Second Foundation of Mindfulness

Once we have some capacity to track and move our attention through the whole field of our sensory, bodily experience, we turn our training to the emotional and mental realms. Now we are not only interested in the pain in our back, but in our interpretation and reaction to the pain. We move from a mindfulness of throbbing to being aware of emotional discomfort and unease. These feelings slip and slide into various flavors, from inevitable disappointment to outright disdain. Just as we have given the physical sensations room to exist or pass without interference, we now allow our emotions room to breathe. This is the second foundation of mindfulness, that of feelings. We may recognize the appearance of utter anxiety or grounded ease; either way, we simply give it our full and unbiased attention, artificially suspending our habits to act out from these emotions.

As we observe our feelings, we inquire into where they live in our bodies, constantly bringing us back to the first foundation of mindfulness, that of the body. We track the interrelationship between our raw sensations and our relationship to those sensations, disentangling them one from the other. Pain is simply pain; pleasure is simply pleasure. These are direct perceptions registered by the brain of unavoidable realities. How we feel and relate to them is a much more subtle and slippery affair of the emotional and mental organism.

To avoid becoming oppressed by or overly identified with what we feel, we must first develop a steady concentration. This is why we begin our training on a simple and unfettered anchor such as the breath. We seldom identify ourselves as being special breathing people, which allows us to relate to the breath with neutrality. Taming our reactivity by developing breath awareness becomes all the more relevant as we progress into mindfulness of emotions and thought patterns. The breath becomes our best ally when we find ourselves lost in the labyrinth of our difficult mind states and in need of a beacon to bring us back. Whether we are bored, depressed, or excited, as we track the various features of these feelings through the body, we keep grounding our capacity to maintain our attention by coming back to the moment-to-moment experience of the breath in the body.

The Third Foundation of Mindfulness

Relaxed concentration teaches us how to relate to ourselves without condemnation or avoidance, but it also allows us to remain with the direct experience as it unfolds, discontinuing our habits of conceptualizing experience and thereby distancing ourselves from the immediacy of life. Over time, we develop the capacity to watch our mental states rise and fall like the breath, without being compelled to believe in or even finish the story line. This is mindfulness of the mind. Whether our thoughts are pearls of profundity or primitive and profane, we can learn to allow them to float though our consciousness as if we are merely writing on water.

Loving-kindness and Compassion. As our mental alertness strengthens, we are encouraged to promote positive mind states while learning to diminish negative ones. The wholesome thoughts we bring to mind and allow to proliferate are those comprising loving-kindness (*metta*) and compassion (*karuna*). In this section of the training, we begin to train the heart through the mind.

There are a number of pithy phrases used in metta and karuna practices. I have selected a few that can be employed for a broad range of support. Traditionally, you begin the training directing these charitable proclamations toward yourself. As courage and self-confidence grow, you embark on the practice of dispatching these fortifying declarations to a host of others. First pick a loved one, then a mentor or benefactor, a neutral person in your life, and eventually your adversaries. The full fruition of this practice cultivates a magnanimous yearning for the welfare of all beings.

You can work with one stanza exclusively when it precisely captures the necessary sentiment, or alternate between them. You can commence your mindful practices with metta or karuna phrases, evoke them midstream (I often recite them during lengthy yoga poses), or allow them to seal each formal session. You may enjoy beginning a practice with these assertions directed toward yourself, and then ending the session by donating them to others. You can even try sitting for an entire metta-based meditation session or go on a retreat emphasizing these themes throughout.

These deceptively simple messages are essential nutrition for the brain, stabilizing and entraining new neural pathways while antidoting habits of disdainful desperation and habitual complacency. Whether you use them ceremoniously or evoke them sporadically throughout the day, consistently saturating the mind with these idioms undeniably refines our quotidian attitudes while forging invaluable pathways to the heart.

Classic metta phrases:

> May I (You) be free of fear and harm.
> May I (You) be content as I am.
> May I (You) be at peace with what comes.

Classic karuna phrases:

> As I experience loneliness (or any difficult emotion), I know others feel this too. May I be willing to open to loneliness with support.
> As you experience loneliness (choosing someone to work with who you know is struggling), I know I have experienced this too. May we both be willing to open to loneliness with support.
> As I experience connectedness (or any emotion of well-being), I know others desire to feel this too. May we all be willing to feel connectedness fully.

The insidious mind states we learn to transform during mindfulness training are greed, hatred, and delusion. The Buddha called them the three poisons because they contaminate our inner life, cunningly obstructing access to our natural benevolence. These profoundly habitual attitudes separate us from our best intentions, expressing them instead through our all-too-familiar negative compulsions and addictions. Learning to listen attentively when these thoughts arise, to disidentify from the often-destructive content of the mind, and to ride the

waves of changing sensations coursing through us, painstakingly heralds new possibilities for us, and is a healing road toward liberating ourselves from suffering.

The Fourth Foundation of Mindfulness

As our attention begins to track ever more subtle aspects of our inner world, we can train in contemplating various objects in our field of attention. This is the fourth foundation of mindfulness. There are many teachings on various subjects for introspection, such as the four noble truths (see page 171), the five hindrances (see page 173), and the six sense doors (i.e., seeing, hearing, tasting, smelling, touching, thinking). Since the fourth foundation is multifaceted, I often isolate one aspect, mindfulness of our environment. The first three foundations all related to our inner world (our sensations, emotions, and thoughts), while the fourth allows us to open up our attention to include sights, sounds, smells, temperature, and so on. This of course brings us back to tracking our sensations, feelings, and thoughts in relation to this external stimuli. With this training, we lose the need to sequester ourselves in quiet vaults of controlled serenity. Instead, we let life happen all around us, watching how we react to the changing features, while suspending our usual compulsion to act out based on our reactions. Whether a sound is brash or melodious, we allow it to be known in the field of our attention, interested in detecting when raw open listening segues into aversion toward a harsh noise or craving for sweet sounds. This aspect of mindfulness allows us to see that the aversion or clinging is not in the thing itself, but within us.

As we learn to relax and open to the contents of our experience, we can begin to explore placing our attention on awareness itself, investigating the nature of our mind. There is a well-known Tibetan story of a young aspirant who goes to his master for further instructions after he has been training in mindfulness for many years. His teacher suggests that instead of tracking his various sensations, emotions, and thoughts, the student must now look for his mind in all his moments of meditation. Enthusiastic that he has been given the next step in his development, the student bounds off to his meditation cave to further his practice. After only a few months, the exasperated seeker is back in front of his teacher feeling despondent.

"When you asked me to follow my breath, I found that after my initial distractions subsided, I was able to track its life cycles with greater and greater ease. When you later expanded your instruction, requesting that I learn to observe all of my many sensations, reactions, and thoughts, I again was able to disentangle the passing inner events from any identification with what was happening, resting in pure observing attention. But now I feel completely defeated, as though all my training has been useless. Whenever I try to find my mind, it eludes me. No matter where I look, I cannot find it anywhere!" Now sobbing and dejected, he begs forgiveness from his master for misrepresenting himself as a worthy vessel for the teachings and rises to leave. The master restrains him at the door. With head bowed, the boy awaits the expected reprimand. Instead, his teacher slowly approaches him with an ironic smile, looks into his eyes, and says, "Very good work. Continue to train like this the rest of your life."

As we patiently expose ourselves over and over to the primordial question of identity, we loosen our conventional identification with our body, emotions and mental states, opening ourselves to an experiential sense of something larger than any of these temporary and changing expressions can define. The insight that we do not actually possess a solid, substantial self that we can find can be quite disorienting initially (although this does not cancel out the unique functioning self we refer to as "me"). Yet if we continue to practice with appropriate support from a qualified teacher, this discovery gradually carves the way for us to loosen our rigidities and see beyond our limiting self-definitions.

20

Mindfulness Meditation

To BEGIN MINDFULNESS TRAINING, you need to be aware of three distinct behaviors. The first is called arriving and centering; the second is anchoring and labeling; and the third is allowing and letting go.

Arriving and Centering

Arriving into a seated mindfulness practice involves body awareness first. Choose a viable sitting posture that feels fairly comfortable for at least 10 minutes. One such posture is often called Burmese Pose. Your feet are placed in front of each other in front of the pelvis; your knees are spread wide and resting down on the floor (Fig. 20.1). You may rest one or both knees on an extra cushion or blanket to help relax your groin muscles and stabilize your knees (Fig. 20.2). If you have chronic back pain, you can sit with your back near a wall and place a soft block

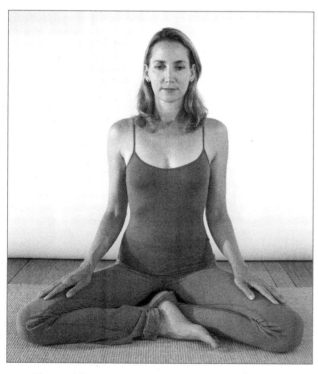

20.1. Burmese Pose

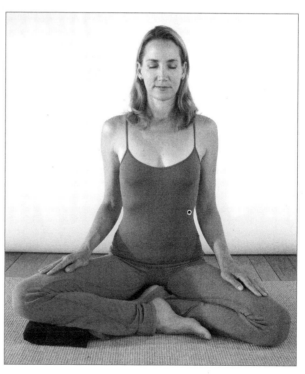

20.2. Burmese Pose, Variation 1

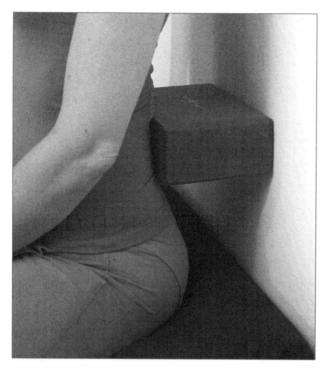

20.3. Burmese Pose, Variation 2

between your lumbar spine and the wall (Fig. 20.3). (If you are bedridden, you can lie on your back, but keep your eyes open so you do not fall asleep.) When sitting, have a cushion or pillow under your sitting bones to maintain a slight tilt forward in the pelvis. This will prevent pressing the weight back into the buttocks, which presses on the sciatic notch and can cause or aggravate sciatica.

Another version of this pose is called Easy Pose (Sukhasana), in which you place each foot under the opposite knee (Fig. 20.4). You can also slip one foot under the opposite ankle (Fig. 20.5), taking Adept's Pose (Siddhasana).

If you have tight outer hips or sciatica, you may want to choose Thunderbolt Pose (Vajrasana) rather than one of the cross-legged poses. Here, you sit with your feet pointing back and your buttocks on a cushion (Fig. 20.6). This naturally tilts your pelvis forward rather than backward, helping

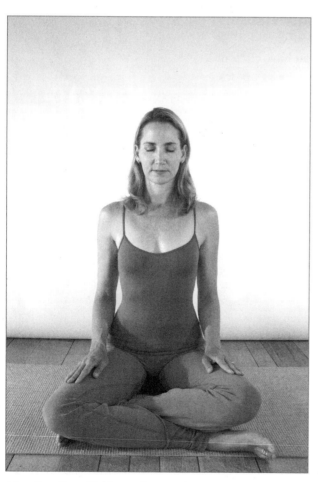

20.4. Easy Pose (Sukhasana)

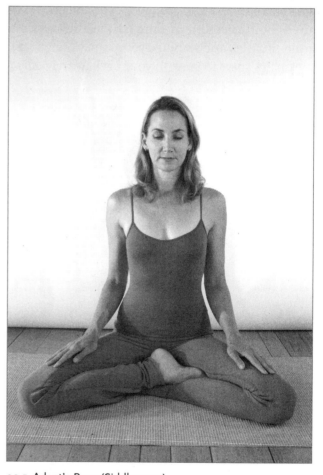

20.5. Adept's Pose (Siddhasana)

maintain the natural arch in your lumbar curve. (Note that you cannot use a block against the wall for support in this posture.)

If you have more external range of motion in your outer hips, you can place one foot on top of the opposite thigh in Half-Lotus Pose (Ardha Padmasana). The sole of your bottom foot rests against the inside of the opposite thigh with your heel near your perineum (Fig. 20.7). If you have very open hips, you can rest each foot on the opposite thigh (Fig. 20.8); this is called Lotus Pose (Padmasana).

Once you have chosen your posture for this practice session, settle into your seat. Lengthen the vertical axis of your spine, allowing the natural curves of your back to remain intact. Join your hands in the center with the thumbs lightly touching each other and the left fingers resting between the knuckles of the right hand. Your intertwined hands can be placed on your thighs or slightly above. Alternately, you can place your hands palms down on your thighs, neither too far

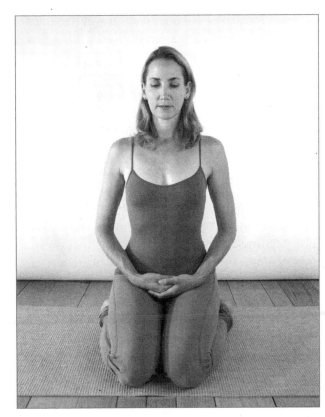

20.6. Thunderbolt Pose (Vajrasana)

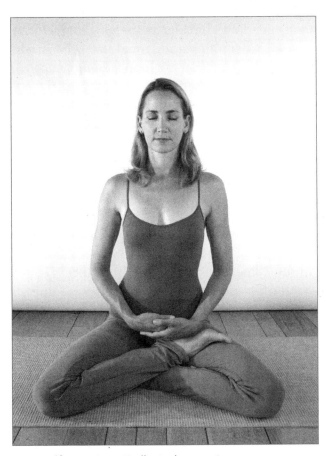

20.7. Half-Lotus Pose (Ardha Padmasana)

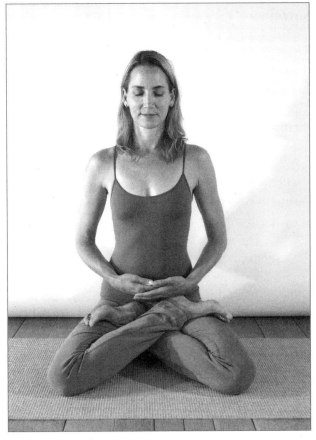

20.8. Lotus Pose (Padmasana)

forward toward your knees (which will misalign you and eventually stress your knees and back as you start to lean forward), nor pulled back near your hips, (which can cause you to unconsciously hike your shoulders up around your ears). When your hands are well placed, you will feel like your elbows hang freely and your shoulders easily rest down your back. Keep your upper torso stacked above your hips, reaching the crown of your head up to kiss the sky. Relax all the muscles in your face, releasing your jaw and allowing your tongue to float freely, neither pressing up on the palate nor pushing down. Lower your gaze or close your eyes almost completely, allowing a tiny sliver of light to penetrate through. You have arrived!

Now that you are situated and aligned, you can center. Begin by committing yourself to staying still now that you are in position (unless, of course, to do so feels risky to any of your joints), even if a cool breeze comes through an open window or you begin to hear voices or noise outside your room. There is no need to maintain special conditions of any kind here, as you are training in opening to every situation without preference.

Centering helps us remember the value of what we are doing now. Reciting a few inspiring lines before we begin is a reminder of the essential value of this practice each time we do it so as not to abandon our intent at the first signs of difficulty or doubt. A few phrases that capture our dedication to practice can help us sift through the often conflicting attitudes we entertain.

I have three phrases that align me each time I begin:

> I vow now to open to awareness for the benefit of all beings.
> I appreciate its immeasurable value.
> I feel it is possible for me in this moment, regardless of conditions and inclusive of all circumstances.

I find that when I reestablish my commitment to pay attention inwardly by vowing to be aware, I remember that this practice benefits not only me, but also all other beings I will encounter as well. Remembering that living with awareness

has immeasurable value relaxes my fixation on all the other things I could choose to do right now, as my attitude will directly affect *everything* I do. Remembering that awareness is possible for me undermines any apathy I may be feeling and reminds me that this is not about some faraway goal in an abstract future. It is about being aware here and now in my personal, verifiable experience, no matter what that is.

Day after day, I have found that the final phrase—"regardless of conditions and inclusive of all circumstances"—is the most important to this vow. It nullifies all excuses, complaints, and distractions. I may be dealing with catastrophic or monumental situations in my personal life, but I can invite them onto the path. With this vow in mind, I take refuge in awareness as a place to come home to throughout all of life's changes.

Anchoring and Labeling

After arriving and centering, you are ready for the main part of practice, the anchoring and labeling. Now it is time to anchor on the breath and then open into a broader awareness that includes sensations, emotions, and mind states. Focused, one-pointed attention is a foundation practice in many styles of meditation and particularly in Buddhist mindfulness. In Buddhism, it is called *shamatha,* meaning "tranquillity" or "calm abidance." The purpose of this initial exclusive focus is to settle down and in, breeding a concentrated state of mind that is both relaxed and alert. Since it is difficult to explore moment-to-moment experience with any consistency when you are easily distracted, this simple practice of resting the attention on a single anchor without seeking any outcome other than pure observance is considered an essential foundation for mindfulness practice.

The method often chosen for developing this one-pointed, calm attention is breath awareness. Resting the attention on the in- and out-breaths is called *anapanasati.* With this method, you do not enhance the breath as in pranayama practices, nor do you forget the breath altogether. You simply rest the mind on the natural movement of each cycle of breathing while relaxing the habit to classify, enhance, or comment on your experience. You can examine the movement of breath as it enters and exits your nostrils, as it makes its way through your whole torso, or as it causes your abdomen to rise and fall. Wherever you choose to watch the breath, this attempt to cultivate a non-interfering attention allows you to see clearly the habits of entanglement that so easily arise in an ordinary moment of living.

Becoming aware of distractions and letting them go is what strengthens concentration. Sometimes you may notice five or six breaths in a row and then suddenly be off—revisiting past experiences, fantasizing about future ones, or compulsively commenting on the present. Other times you may be absolutely unaware in your body or mind, and your moments pass in a fuzzy haze of spaciness.

I remember hearing the story of a man who had the habit of sitting down with a firm intention to pay attention to his breath and meditate but would inevitably find himself standing in front of the open refrigerator. This kind of absent-mindedness is actually the opposite of mindfulness. We are often led around by our impulses and compulsions, our uninvestigated conditioning, unaware of how our whole organism is directed from unconscious patterns of mind (or belly). The shamatha practice allows us to witness these strong patterns of behavior in the clear light of awareness, without judgment or expectation. With practice, these inebriated mental lapses are shortened and even lose their power of seduction. The mind begins to enjoy resting in its natural state of calm attention.

As you sit and attempt to track your inhalations and exhalations, you may find your discursive mind so frustratingly unwieldy that you need to use thinking to train your mind. You can use any of four different shamatha tools in these instances. The first is counting. As you inhale, count one and then simply listen to the exhalation. As you inhale again, count two, and so on. When you have gone all the way to ten, rest again without counting on the sound and feel of the breath. If you get distracted before ten, start again at one. If you make it to ten and still feel unable to stay with the breath, inhale and count nine, exhale quietly, inhale and count eight, and so on, all the way down to one again. This can continue, if necessary, back up to eight and then down to one, up to seven and then down, and so forth. Eventually (if not in this session, then in a future one), the mind will relinquish its wild ways and settle; it is the nature of cause and effect.

Another effective concentration method is to inhale and say to yourself, "Inhaling I am just here now"; and as you exhale say, "exhaling I am releasing resistance." Then rest in the silence that echoes after these promptings. When you get distracted again, repeat the lines with breathing as often as you need to.

A third way to relax with the breath is to engender some loving-kindness toward yourself as well as sending it out to others. Inwardly you can say, "Inhaling may I be at peace; exhaling may all feel peace," while you breathe. After this, rest in the silent space of inner listening, coming back to the saying again as soon as you notice that you have drifted away from breath awareness.

A fourth method is nonconceptual. Simply watching the unique event of each breath cycle, you track the beginning, middle, and end of the inhalation, then myopically focus on the beginning, middle, and end of the exhalation. Whether the breath is long or short, deep or shallow, listen to each with interest as if it is the only one you will ever take. Studying the breath in this way, you can observe the constant cycles of pleasant, neutral, and unpleasant feelings that occur naturally with the breathing process. As you begin to breathe in, you feel good taking in a new supply of oxygen. As you continue to inhale, you begin to take it for granted that you are able to breathe fully, so the feeling is neutral. As the inhalation finishes and you are filled to capacity, you notice that it becomes unpleasant the longer you hold the breath. But as soon as the exhalation begins, you feel pleasure again, and the cycle repeats itself over and over. As you observe the natural tides of breath, you garner insight into the constant fluctuations of pleasant, neutral, and unpleasant feelings that are intrinsic to all experiences. Over time, this realization can diminish attempts to promote only the pleasant or to feel somehow defeated whenever the unpleasant arises.

These four ways of focusing on the breath appeal to different people depending on their character or can each be used by the same person depending on your needs at the time. Even when you have a style you find comfortable, inevitable distractions will arise, but you need not find them worrisome. They are natural tendencies of the un-trained mind and can be sympathetically worked with rather than resented.

Once you have arrived and centered on the breath (and later sensations, feelings, mind states, and environmental stimuli), you can settle into the heart of the practice by anchoring and labeling. Almost immediately, your attention will want to wander off. No need to despair, as this is to be expected. You are seeing how compelling it is for your concentration to jump from this ob-ject to anything else. Rather than berate yourself, mindfulness training expands on breath aware-ness and begins to allow any "distraction" to be known directly as it is.

As I sat the other morning gazing out the win-dow, I heard my fourteen-year-old daughter come into the room. I invited her to come sit in my lap like she used to when she was little, silently sucking her thumb while I stayed in mindful-ness practice. She plopped her big, warm body into my lap, saying, "But I don't know how to meditate." I told her it wasn't something she had to be taught; it was the most natural thing in the world, and she did it all the time. Upon hearing this, her body seemed to settle into me, and our breathing synchronized as she sat looking out the window with me. When we both noticed a bright blue hummingbird suckling a lovely crimson flower, my daughter silently pointed her finger. I named the event out loud: "seeing." A few quiet moments passed before she shifted her weight, and I said, "Discomfort." Next her stomach growled, and I whispered, "Hunger." She whis-pered back, "I want you to make me breakfast," and I noted, "Craving." She laughed, jumped up, and tried pulling me off the floor while I yelled, "Resistance, resistance!" We had effortlessly sat in mindfulness for more than ten minutes, just experiencing the changing nature of phenomena while living from the stable center of attention. This is mindfulness practice.

During such practice, you sit committed to watching the breath, while life unfolds in its natu-ral way; you simply track and label the changing features, coming back to the breath as soon as you have noted whatever else has arisen. As your practice matures, you can allow your anchor to shift from the breath to sensations in your body, watching all the other manifestations arise and fall, while returning again and again to your cur-rent physical feelings. The same can be done with emotions, mind states, and even sounds in your environment as your anchor. The inclusion of these various features is the practice of the four foundations of mindfulness.

Whether you focus on changing sensations or mind states, you will wake up to the wandering mind by labeling where you go. Use the simplest one-word description to help you wake up to what has pulled your attention. While the five hin-drances will be the distractions you notice most often, you can particularize the labels in each area of experience. *Throbbing, pinching, tickling, sweat-ing,* and *shivering* are common for sensations; *uneasy, disappointed, joyous,* and *resentful* might illustrate emotions; and *waiting, judging, plan-ning,* and *dreading* are descriptions of mind states. Once you have noted what is occurring and whis-pered this label to yourself, immediately return to the object of meditative attention.

Accepting and Letting Go

Two attitudes can help you maintain the alert aliveness you are developing; they are accepting and letting go. While you practice mindfulness, you temporarily suspend your tendency to edit or censure what is happening. This means that if you want to be mindful, you have to accept what mindfulness finds. Say "yes" to your entire experience as it occurs, and allow each feature to come and go within the field of your attention. As you engender an atmosphere of allowance, you also let go of your habitual assumptions about what you think should be happening in contrast to what actually is. You are not, for example, try-ing to let go of the pain in your hip; instead, you are letting go of thinking that your hip should feel different, while also letting go of resisting the pain. You can imagine you are behaving like a tree in the forest that does not wrestle with the heat or the pounding rain, push away a bird's nest, or scratch at the crawling insects. You are allowing and letting be in equanimity.

Once you are able to track the arising and passing of phenomena with some stability, you are ready for insight practice, or vipassana. Your mindful attention now investigates the nature of its object, exploring the three characteristics of all conditioned things—anicca, dukkha, and anatta. Now you not only know that your knee throbs or your mind doubts, but you look into how this sensation or thought is configured, meaning its essence. You literally inquire into its seeming solidity and stability. Through your moment-to-moment investigation of each detail, you can discover that even something as pervasive as pain fluctuates constantly. Under closer scrutiny, you see solid realities break up into undulating oscillations that are not at all stable. This is insight into the impermanence of all objects (anicca). When you ignore this fact and find that you are clinging to or resisting what is occuring, you experience and investigate dukkha (unsatisfactoriness), becoming aware of its insubstantiality as well.

As you continue to examine your objects of attention, you continue to question their isolated, separate existence. This investigation leads you to see how contingent all experience is. You see how a thought arises out of a memory, which arose out of a past experience that arose out of many factors coming together, which could only occur because of many former things coalescing, and so on. At this stage of practice, you see the empty nature of phenomena; how all things are mutually dependent and empty of permanent self-existence—in other words, selfless (anatta).

As you sit and watch the breath, you are now open to the full matrix of your experience. You may notice a jabbing sensation in your back (the first foundation), an obvious feeling of discomfort (the second foundation), a willingness to watch it fluctuate and pulsate (the third foundation). After a while, you hear a door slam (the fourth foundation) and then notice resistance to the discomfort vibrating again in your back (dukkha and aversion). A voice says, "I can't stand this another moment," then inquires, "Who can't stand this?" (investigation into the solid sense of "me," anatta and the third foundation). As you search for this phantom, you may notice the flowing, breathing body and come back to simple breath awareness, ready to turn toward whatever happens next. This training is a cultivation of open readiness, and each session, each moment will be different. Paying attention with clarity and interest eventually negates the common description of anything being boring, as you are now breeding the possibility of intimacy with your direct experience, whatever that may be. You are diminishing your harmony addiction and instead learning to adapt rather than fight or collapse within any situation.

Although you set aside special time to cultivate mindful attention, either in sitting or in Yin postures, the real training begins when you leave the cushion. The Buddha was once asked what the most important moment in practice is, and he said, "The moment you get up!" As you end each formal practice, your main interest is in translating this radical presence into the many activities of your day. The best way to accomplish this is to end the session by dedicating the merit of the practice to the benefit of others and then generating gratitude for those who inspire you, vowing to them to sustain your interest in aware living. I do this by bringing to mind someone I am close to and who I know is currently struggling with some life situation.

To do this, imagine such a person seated in front of you; you begin to breathe in and out harmoniously together. On the inhalation, empathize with her pain and recite, "I feel how difficult this is for you." On the exhalation, say, "May you feel my support." After a number of breaths, imagine that this person is joined by thousands of people who are suffering in a similar way and that you send them the same wishes, "May you all feel supported and find relief from your suffering." This attitude of caring can then be turned toward your teachers. Send them wishes for a long, healthy life (if they are still alive) and/or wish that they will continue to positively influence many others. Imagine your teachers gathered around you, seated in a circle of support, creating a personal mandala (sacred circle) with you in the center. In their presence, end the session with a renewed commitment to open to awareness for the benefit of all beings, just as you did when you began your practice. Ending with a bow, repeat, "May all beings find true freedom in whatever way is available to them."

Whether you start this path of awareness as a formal sitting practice or as part of a Yin yoga practice, the main point is to learn to extend mindfulness into all your activities and relationships—from performing active yoga asanas to parenting, from running errands to relating to others. There is no corner of life that need be excluded from the path of awareness. This means that your life is not in the way; the way is to be lived through your life! As you begin to drop the war with what is and breed insight into its nature, you create the possibility of a new way of being, one that leads you away from suffering and directly toward true happiness.

Namaste.

Appendix

Sequencing Notes

SEQUENCING IS A VERY PERSONAL ART, but I would like to share
some guidelines that I have found helpful. On most days, I begin with
the nine clearing cycles and then with meditation and then move into the
Yin practice (short or long, depending on my schedule), often alternating
the Kidney sequence (see page 48) with the Liver sequence (see page 66).
Then some days, especially if I am teaching a lot of hours that day or going
hiking, I move through the Sun Salutation (Surya Namaskar) sequence
and then take Corpse Pose (Savasana). On other days, when I know I will
be less physical, I alternate the Practice for Stimulating the Kidneys and
Circulating Yang Chi to the Core (see page 136) with the Fire-Building
Yang Practice (see page 148) before the final relaxation.

If I am experiencing an abundance of agitation, irritation, or restlessness, I practice the Liver sequence. I also choose this sequence when I
want to feel more space in my hips for meditation or when my body has
had to digest more toxins than usual.

When I am feeling somewhat apprehensive or confused, scared or
fearful, I do the Kidney session. I also engage in this sequence when I
am feeling less inner moisture or when my energy is particularly low,
as the body is continually drawing from the kidney chi to boost any energy depletion.

On days when I am on the computer a lot, I make sure to incorporate the Yang sessions, while active days in the city send me more toward the Yin practices for balance.

Whenever I am under the weather, on my moon cycle, healing from
any illness, enduring really hot weather, experiencing an abundance
of inner heat, or just feeling somewhat stressed and overburdened, I
gravitate toward a Yin practice with an emphasis on the kidneys—one
in the morning and/or one in the late afternoon.

Although on most days I incorporate meditation with Yin poses
and then Yang, there are variations I sometimes apply. For instance,
some days I find meditating and doing a Yang practice in the morning
is complemented by a Yin session in the evening before dinner. If my
day is too full for much practice, I simply begin with meditation and
come into a Yin practice before going to sleep at night.

On days when I need to have a lot of energy and mental focus, I begin with meditation and then the Yin style, often coming into the Yang

practice at the end of the day to wash away the intensity of my day, refreshing my vibrancy before evening. When my life has a balance of activity and rest and I do not have enough time for Yin and Yang practices each day, I tend to alternate them, doing meditation and Yin yoga one day, meditation and a Yang practice the next.

Obviously, it is important to acknowledge the many factors going on in our day, coupled with what is going on inside us, in order to create the appropriate combinations of sequences to encourage balance.

To begin to trust your own ability to guide your practice authentically, take a few minutes before beginning each day to intuit which sequences you think will help you cultivate vibrant energy, an open heart, and a clear and spacious mind. Later in the day reflect on whether these qualities were indeed enhanced in your experience, and adjust your next day's practice accordingly. This will help you continue to keep your practice flexible and integral, as well as interesting, fresh, and alive.

Suggestions for Sequences

Various sequences can be joined together with the Yin, Yang, pranayama and mindfulness practices, creating different effects in our body-mind experience. For example, when we begin with meditation, it allows us to move into everything that follows from an inward-drawn, connected place. When we end with meditation, the various asana practices prepare the body-mind effectively for this stillness discipline.

In general, all the sequences are designed to draw our focus inward, but each will likely have a different effect on every person. I have provided some information in the following list to show how these sessions may affect you, but please listen to your own experience and allow that to be your best guide on how and when to combine these practices.

- Yang for beginners sequence, Corpse Pose (Savasana), and meditation (10 minutes): Good if you are new to yoga or to these practices
- Yin Kidney sequence, Sun Salutation (Surya Namaskar) with variations, Corpse Pose (Savasana), pranayama, meditation (10 to 20 minutes): Balances fear and/or lack of inspiration, as well as energy depletion
- Nine clearing cycles, meditation (15 minutes), Yin Liver sequence, Yang core sequence, and Corpse Pose (Savasana): Balances anger, resentment, physical toxicity, and lethargy
- Yin Liver sequence, Sun Salutation (Surya Namaskar) without variations, Corpse Pose (Savasana), and pranayama meditation (20 minutes): Balances frustration, moodiness, and fatigue
- Nine clearing cycles, meditation (20 minutes), Kidney Yin sequence, Fire-Building Yang sequence, and Corpse Pose (Savasana): Balances disconnectedness, spaciness, sedentariness, and computer haze

- Kidney Yin sequence, Corpse Pose (Savasana), and meditation (10 minutes): Balances sickness, weakness, and a fragile immune system
- Nine clearing cycles, Sun Salutation (Surya Namaskar) with variations, Corpse Pose (Savasana), pranayama, and meditation (15 minutes): Balances excess mental stimulation
- Meditation (10 minutes), Yang core sequence, and Corpse Pose (Savasana): Balances hypertension and encourages freshness
- Stomach/Spleen Yin sequence, Sun Salutation (Surya Namaskar) without variations, Corpse Pose (Savasana), pranayama, and meditation (20 minutes): Balances anxiety, purposelessness, and self-doubt
- Meditation (10 minutes), Lung/Heart/Intestine Yin sequence, Corpse Pose (Savasana), pranayama, and meditation: Balances grief, despair, obsession, and feelings of being under the weather
- Nine clearing cycles, meditation (10 minutes), Stomach/Spleen Yin sequence, meditation (20 minutes): Balances indigestion, cramps, worry, and overthinking
- Liver Yin sequence, pranayama, and meditation (15 minutes): Balances edginess, frustration, and discontent

Suggested Readings

B ELOW I HAVE LISTED some resources to deepen your understanding of the subjects in this book. For a more detailed book list please visit my website, http://sarahpowers.com.

Books on Taoism and Chinese Medicine

Beinfield, Harriet, and Efrem Korn. *Between Heaven and Earth: A Guide to Chinese Medicine.* New York: Ballantine Books, 1992.

Chia, Mantak, and Maneewan Chia. *Awaken Healing Light of the Tao.* Huntington, N.Y.: Healing Tao Books, 1993.

Grilley, Paul. *Yin Yoga: Outline of a Quiet Practice.* Ashland, Ore.: White Cloud Press, 2002.

Johnson, Larry. *Yoga Alchemy.* Crestone, Colo.: White Elephant Monastery, 2004.

Kaptchuk, Ted. *The Web That Has No Weaver.* New York: Contemporary Books, 2000.

Motoyama, Hiroshi. *Awakening the Chakras and Emancipation.* Tokyo: Human Science Press, 2003.

———. *Theories of the Chakras: Bridge to Higher Consciousness.* Wheaton, Ill.: Theosophical Publishing House, 1981.

———. *Toward a Superconciousness: Meditational Theory and Practice.* Translated by Shigenori Nagatomo and Clifford R. Ames. Berkeley, Calif.: Asian Humanities Press, 1990.

Books on Yoga

Cope, Stephen. *The Wisdom of Yoga: A Seeker's Guide to Extraordinary Living.* New York: Bantam Dell, 2006.

Desikachar, T. K. V. *The Heart of Yoga: Developing a Personal Practice.* Rochester, Vt.: Inner Traditions International, 1995.

Iyengar, B. K. S. *Light on Yoga.* New York: Schocken Books, 1966.

Kraftsow, Gary. *Yoga for Wellness.* New York: Penguin Group, 1999.

Kramer, Joel. *The Passionate Mind: A Manual for Living Creatively with One's Self.* Berkeley, Calif.: North Atlantic Books, 1974.

Lasater, Judith. *Living Your Yoga.* Berkeley, Calif.: Rodmell Press, 1999.

Rosen, Richard. *Pranayama: Beyond the Fundamentals.* Boston, Mass.: Shambhala Publications, 2006.

Schiffmann, Erich. *The Spirit and Practice of Moving into Stillness.* New York: Pocket Books, 1996.

Swatmarama, Yogi. *Hatha Yoga Pradapika.* Translated by Swami Muktibodhananda Saraswati. Bihar, India: Bihar School of Yoga, 1985.

Books on Buddhism

Batchelor, Stephen. *Buddhism Without Beliefs.* New York: Riverhead Books, 1997.

Brach, Tara. *Radical Acceptance: Embracing Your Life with the Heart of a Buddha.* New York: Bantam Dell, 2003.

Gunaratana, Bhante. *Mindfulness in Plain English.* Somerville, Mass.: Wisdom Publications, 2002.

Kornfield, Jack. *A Path with Heart.* New York: Bantam Books, 1993.

McLeod, Ken. *Wake Up to Your Life: Discovering the Buddhist Path to Attention.* New York: HarperCollins, 2001.

Rosenberg, Larry. *Breath by Breath: The Liberating Practice of Insight Meditation.* Boston, Mass.: Shambhala Publications, 1998.

Salzberg, Sharon. *Lovingkindness: The Revolutionary Art of Happiness.* Boston, Mass.: Shambhala Publications, 1995.

Silananda, U. *The Four Foundations of Mindfulness.* Somerville, Mass.: Wisdom Publications, 2002.

Smith, Jean. *The Beginner's Guide to Walking the Buddha's Eightfold Path.* Somerville, Mass.: Wisdom Publications, 2002.

Thakar, Vimala. *Why Meditation.* Delhi, India: Motilal Banarsidass Publishers, 1977.

Welwood, John. *Toward a Psychology of Awakening: Buddhism, Psychotherapy, and the Path of Personal and Spiritual Transformation.* Boston, Mass.: Shambhala Publications, 2000.

Acknowledgments

As we all know, every project is a collective effort, and I have many people to thank for helping bring this one to fruition. First of all, I want to express my deep appreciation to Linda Sparrowe, who not only encouraged me to write this book but also spent many afternoons with me helping me become a better writer. Linda and Richard Rosen introduced me to Emily Bower, who has been the best editor I could have imagined. I want to express my deepest gratitude to Paul Grilley for contributing an eloquent foreword and for being such a superior teacher, a dedicated friend, and an example of genuine integrity in my life. I also feel so grateful to have been able to work with the photographer Matthew Carden, who did such lovely photographs and worked exhausting hours adding the meridians to many of the photos. He was the one who sped me along after years of writing in fits and starts by suggesting we do this project together.

I also want to thank my wonderful friend and shining assistant, Doran Christie, who introduced me to my illustrator, Kathi Tesarz, who I want to thank for her clear drawings done in such a timely manner. I am also indebted to my sweet friend Kathryn Arnold, who was the first one to read the first draft and who gave me such heartfelt encouragement and direction for how to proceed. I also want to thank the many teachers who have influenced this synthesis of subjects, including Tsoknyi Rinpoche, Jennifer Welwood, Tsultrim Allione, Bhante Gunaratana, Stephen and Martine Batchelor, Jack Kornfield, S. N. Goenka, Dr. Hiroshi Motoyama, Sri Krishnamacharya, B. K. S. Iyengar, T. K.V. Desikachar, Gary Kraftsow, Richard Freeman, Erich Schiffmann, Joel Kramer, Ana Forrest, Chuck Miller, Aadil Palkhivala, Ted Kaptchuck, Mantak Chia, Larry Johnson, and too many more to name. Most of all, I want to thank my daughter, Imani Jade, for being such a jewel in my life and my generous and insightful husband, Ty Powers, who helped me clarify all these subjects through our many hours of discussion and inquiry, reading and revisioning this manuscript, and who is such a bright light for many of us.

Index of Yoga Poses

Yin Poses

Yang Poses